Teenage Cancer Journey

By Kathleen A. Gill

With illustrations by Allison A. Hicks

Oncology Nursing Press, Inc.
A subsidiary of the Oncology Nursing Society
Pittsburgh, PA

Oncology Nursing Press, Inc.

Publisher: Leonard Mafrica, MBA
Technical Publications Editor: Barbara Sigler, RN, MNEd
Staff Editor: Lisa M. George, BA
Creative Services Assistants: Chad Chronick, Dany Sjoen

Teenage Cancer Journey

Library of Congress Catalog Card Number: 99-068910

ISBN 1-890504-13-0

Publisher's Note

This book is published by the Oncology Nursing Press, Inc. (ONP). ONP neither represents nor guarantees that the practices described herein will, if followed, ensure safe and effective patient care. The recommendations contained in this book reflect ONP's judgment regarding the state of general knowledge and practice in the field as of the date of publication. The recommendations may not be appropriate for use in all circumstances. Those who use this book should make their own determinations regarding specific safe and appropriate patient-care practices, taking into account the personnel, equipment, and practices available at the hospital or other facility at which they are located. The author and publisher cannot be held responsible for any liability incurred as a consequence of the use or application of any of the contents of this book. Mention of specific products and opinions related to those products do not indicate or imply endorsement by ONS or ONP.

ONS and ONP publications are originally published in English. Permission has been granted by the ONS Board of Directors for foreign translation. (Individual tables and figures that are reprinted or adapted require additional permission from the original source.) However, because translations from English may not always be accurate and precise, ONS and ONP disclaim any responsibility for inaccurate translations. Readers relying on precise information should check the original English version.

Printed in the United States of America

Oncology Nursing Press, Inc.
A subsidiary of the Oncology Nursing Society

This book is dedicated with love to Sally Gill, Ted Gordon, Kimberly LaForet, and

Thomas Lenahan. You have taught me the true meaning of courage.

Table of Contents

Foreword

Dear Reader:

Hi. I want to make something clear from the start—I do not die at the end of this book. People of all ages (including me, including teenagers) can and do recover from cancer and go on to lead long, productive, and healthy lives. Cancer is not an automatic death sentence—although on some days I'll admit it felt like one.

There were many times when I thought I was going to die. However, as I'm reminded daily, sometimes what I think is going to happen to me and what really happens to me are two different things.

Three months before my 16th birthday, I was diagnosed with Hodgkin's disease. Cancer. It seemed so unreal. It was as if I stepped outside of my body and, against my will, became trapped in a horror movie. I watched someone else play me, yet knew that I was that someone else and there was no way out.

I left my old life, my "before-cancer" life, and entered this new life, the cancer life. The new life consisted of pain, fear, uncertainty, and sickness. I felt isolated and alone. I felt like the only 15-year-old in the entire universe with cancer. I did not know anyone who had cancer. I wanted to see or touch someone who had cancer and lived to tell about it.

And then one day the phone rang.

It was a young woman who had been in remission from Hodgkin's disease for a few years (her mother-in-law worked with my mother). Her phone call spawned so many conflicting emotions. I was overjoyed to hear from someone who beat cancer as a teenager, especially someone who had the same type of cancer I had. And yet, at the same time, I was jealous of her health. During the 15 months that I was in treatment, her phone call was the only "direct" contact I had with someone who had experienced cancer as a teenager.

When I was at the hospital, I was always interested in the other adolescents who were undergoing cancer treatment. I never sought them out directly, but rather asked my doctor and the pediatric social worker about them. I can't really explain why, but I wasn't ready for face-to-face contact.

I made several visits to the library, searching for materials about teenagers and cancer. This seemed like a safer option. I wanted to read stories about other teenagers with cancer—how they coped, survived, and went on with their lives. I couldn't find anything.

It wasn't until January 1, 1998, after seven-and-a-half years in remission, that I had a telephone conversation with another survivor of teenage cancer. Maria is a survivor of leukemia. She was diagnosed when she was 13 and was nearly 20 when we first spoke. I felt like I had found a long-lost friend, someone whom I'd never met yet who truly understood and related to what I was saying.

The *Teenage Cancer Journey* grew out of a need not only to address cancer in the young adult, but also to talk about the issues that adolescents with cancer must face. I know that each person with cancer has a unique experience, but I feel that there is a point where some experiences and situations are common.

A wise person once told me a story: Jack and Roger, two friends, go out to dinner at a restaurant and have a nice time. The next time Jack and Roger go out to that same restaurant, there is no way that their experience can be exactly the same as it was the previous time. The first experience could be not as good as the second in some ways but was better in other ways, and vice versa. Both situations are different in their own ways and still share some common elements. I believe that so, too, are teenage cancer experiences.

I soon found that the "after-cancer" me needed to write this book. For so long I was living in "cruise-control mode." I just went from here to there, never stopping to brake. I used to think that I could make myself forget about having cancer. I was wrong. And maybe that's not such a bad thing. Anyway, sooner or later we all need to brake and take control again. This book helped me to do that.

I hope this book helps those in the medical community who treat adolescents with cancer to come to a more complete understanding that teenagers are lingering somewhere out there between pediatric and adult oncology.

Lastly, it is my greatest wish that this book will help other teenage patients with cancer and their families to see that they are not alone and that cancer can be survived.

Katie Gill

Acknowledgments

Each time I read a book, I scan through the acknowledgments. As I do, I realize that books usually are not written by the one person or people listed after the word "by" on the front cover. That also is the case with this book, which includes the collective thoughts and stories of many others.

As a result, there are so many special people who I wish to thank for this book's existence.

First and foremost, I thank Dr. David Klooster, my Advanced Writing professor at John Carroll University in Cleveland, OH. He is the reason that this book exists. He went above and beyond the call of duty as my teacher, spending hours of his own time helping me to organize, draft, revise, and edit the copy. But most importantly, he listened to what I had to say about my vision for the book. His belief in this book and in my ability to write it were a constant source of encouragement. He has taught me an invaluable lesson about being a teacher: Great teachers never just teach—they inspire.

My parents, Tom and Karen Gill, always have been there for me. I thank them for their unconditional love and support. Words are inadequate to describe how much they mean to me. My brothers, Tim and Pat, made me tough early. Mom always said we'd wake up one day and find out that we really did like one another. She was right. And Pat, the cartoons you drew are superb. Thanks.

I have been blessed with wonderful friends who have stuck by me and supported me no matter what the weather—and there have been some big storms. Thanks to Kirsten Schnabel, Annmarie LaForet, Liz Szentendrei, Rachel Clark, Tracie Gordon, Amy Brooks, Robin Bobal, Gina Haylash, Norma Salem, Heather Bowers, Akiko Sekine, Carol Dolovacky, Jennifer Couts, Rachel San Jose, and Allison Hicks (artist *extraordinaire*—thanks for all the hard work and great pictures, Ali!). I love ya, girls!

I wish to thank the faculty and staff of Magnificat High School for helping me fulfill my goal of graduating with my class. Thank you for not allowing me to quit and for not lowering your expectations of me.

At John Carroll University, I also wish to thank Dr. Linda Seward, my former teacher and now friend.

Each day, I have the pleasure of learning how to teach by working with the best mentor-teacher, class, and staff around. I wish to thank Thea Sako, my 23 students in Grade 4, Room 3, and the staff at Rowland School. You're the best.

I'd like to thank the Moore family—Tom, Shirley, Jay, Laura, and Miriam. They came into my life at a difficult time, and we had fun.

There are so many people to thank for trusting me enough to send personal accounts of their cancer experiences. It is their wish to help others. Although I have never met most of them, I feel that we have an understood friendship. Thanks to Jane Beckett, Bethany Columbus, Dianne Chapman, Heidi Barone Sanford, Nikki Mosier, Julia Ryan, Susie Johnston, Troy Braden, Amanda Dolezal, Brett Wilson, Marc Dewey, Sam Frost, Kimberley Hagood, Andrea Richardson, Dominic Ramsey, Jim Keefe, Maria Valarezo, Adam Kabel, Annalee Tan, Barbara Cuccovia, Jennifer McFerrin, Amity Cordell, Christine Mizen, and Marshall Buckley.

Thanks to Father Robert Welsh, SJ, Father Dan Reim, SJ, Dr. David Paul, Dr. Michael Levien, Dr. Elizabeth Danish, Lynna Metrisin, and Jeffrey Paul for taking the time to sit down and talk with me. Your insights are central to this book.

Thanks to Melba Joelin Valarezo, Melba M. Valarezo, and Matthew Buckley for having the courage to share what it's like to love someone with cancer.

Brian Devine, thanks for providing such great artwork in a short amount of time. I appreciate it.

Introduction: The Journey

I have this recurring nightmare, or dream, depending on the way I choose to look at it. It started shortly after I was told that I had cancer. Well actually, it started before that. It started when I first felt "the lumps" in my neck, before I was even diagnosed with cancer. It was like my unconscious mind knew that my physical body was in terrible trouble and was trying to let me in on it. Somehow, I just knew something wasn't right.

In my nightmare, I am dead (okay, so now you're probably thinking, Great introduction, Katie). I am in this tacky white casket with an equally tacky brass rim around it. (These details added to the nightmare part.) I am wearing a dress I bought for a dance during my sophomore year of high school. I remember the day I got that dress as if I had purchased it five minutes ago.

"Mom, isn't this dress beautiful?" I asked, grabbing her hand and dragging her over to where the dress hung.

It stuck out. It's a black (how appropriate), short-sleeve, knee-length deal. The top part is solid black and tightly fitted, with six gold buttons. The dress loosens around the waist, giving way to black and purple folds that complete it.

I tried it on in the dressing room. As I stood in front of the mirror, I surveyed myself, starting at the bottom of the dress and slowly moving my gaze upwards, desperately trying to block out my face. From the neck down, I felt that all of my other cancer scars could be adequately covered with clothing, but from the neck up, I felt cruelly betrayed and humiliated. I had dark circles under my eyes. My cheeks looked like they were storing nuts for the winter. My hair was pretty much gone.

And there I stood, wearing a green Boston Celtics' baseball cap and a formal dress.

It was hot and stuffy in the dressing room, but as I came face-to-face with myself in the mirror, a chill went through my body. This itty-bitty voice inside my head whispered, "I wonder if they'll bury you in it?"

Now, any rational person probably would have thrown the dress somewhere and gone running. Me? I got the dress. I don't know why.

That voice and thought haunted me often. I hid the dress in the back of my closet and made mental notes to tell my mom that under no circumstances should I be buried in that dress.

Getting back to the dream, friends and family are standing around my coffin, crying. I see it all so vividly. Their faces are stained red with tears. Their clothes are bright and alive with color. Their skin is pink, alive, full of life. My face is ashen, dead, lifeless. Off to the right is a bulletin board covered with pictures that mark significant moments in my life. Baby pictures. Katie and her first two-wheeled bicycle. It's a bright yellow "Daisy Flower." My parents got it for me because I stopped sucking my thumb.

"I'm never going to suck my thumb again," I proclaimed to all who would listen.

The day I got "Daisy Flower," I rode her up and down the street. That night after "Daisy Flower" was in the garage and I was tucked in my bed, that darned thumb somehow found its way back into my mouth. Racked with guilt and unable to sleep, I wandered downstairs and tearfully confessed to my parents. It amazes me how simple things used to be and yet how terrible they seemed at the time.

School pictures. Various birthday parties. They stop abruptly after my freshman year of high school, right after my cancer diagnosis. I usually forced myself awake at this point and repeated over and over, "It's okay, you're alive. You're okay, you're alive, really you are." Sometimes my face was wet with tears and my body was covered with sweat.

I, to this day, still have this vision. The image of me in the casket is faded, and I don't really see all the people as clearly as before. What I see are the new pictures. Katie graduates from high school and college. She gets her first car. Katie is standing outside the door to her first apartment.

By the way, I decided to wear the "death dress" to my graduation from college. It was so hot that day that I'm surprised I didn't sweat to death in it!

The scenario doesn't scare me anymore. I don't awaken suddenly; in fact, it doesn't wake me up at all. Until recently, I've looked at my life as having two separate parts that are so different that they couldn't possibly form a whole: part one is before cancer, and part two is during and after cancer. I wonder if someday they will somehow blend together and become one. When I turn 30, I'll have lived half of my life prior to diagnosis and the other half post diagnosis. Maybe I'm trying to figure out what role cancer does or did play in my life. Right now, these lives still seem separate.

I really thought I was going to die. I say this not because I am a pessimist, but because I couldn't imagine beating cancer and going on to graduate from high school and college and then go on to graduate school. But I did. I couldn't imagine turning 20 because 20 was "so old." But I did (and by the way, I don't think 20 is all that old anymore). I couldn't imagine ever feeling "not sick" again. But I do.

My doctor asked me a few years ago, "How has cancer changed your life?" He sort of stumped me on that one. I've been thinking about it for a long time, and sometimes when I'm angry or frustrated, it's easy to give an answer like, "I'm scared of relapsing. I walk with a limp, and before I didn't." I think maybe the better answers are the ones that don't come so easily. I would hate to think that I went through all of this and haven't come away with anything positive. I used to like easy answers—black and white, right or wrong. Cancer is like an option on a true-or-false test, the ones that read "all of the following are true except," for which there are subtle shades of gray.

One thing is for absolute certain: I'd go through it all again if I had to. I'd do it all again because being able to live is worth it all.

Chapter 1.

From Diagnosis
Through Remission

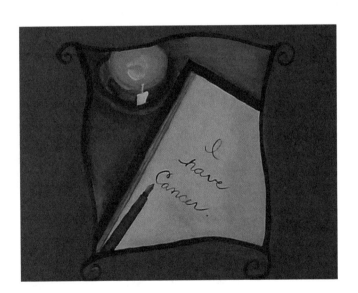

Chapter 1.

From Diagnosis Through Remission

How It All Began

I didn't have a phone in my bedroom, so I was in my parents' bedroom, sprawled across their bed and so twisted up in the phone cord that I had to pull on it to get the receiver to my ear. The voice on the other end asked, "Did you have fun at the Valentine's Day dance?"

"Yeah, I guess," I replied. Actually, I thought it was boring. The previous week, all of the girls in my seventh-grade class, myself included, had been agonizing over what we were going to wear and where we were going to eat before the dance. And when Friday night finally came along, the first slow song of the night sent everyone into a panic. The girls moved to one side of the gym and the boys to the other. We just stood there, all dressed up, looking at each other and thinking, What do we do now?

There were a few exceptions. Two couples ventured out onto the dance floor. And several pairs of eyes stared with shy envy as they started to dance. After what seemed like a time equal to two school years, the disc jockey played a fast song, and it seemed as if everyone let out a collective deep breath and became themselves again.

Sensing that my friend on the other line had similar feelings about what was supposed to be the biggest social moment in our seventh-grade lives, I asked, "So, did you have a good time?"

"Yeah, I think so," she said.

My friend then mentioned that she had been to see her dentist the very Friday of the dance, and he said she was coming down with a cold. "How can your dentist figure out if you are coming down with a cold?" I asked, figuring she was just trying to come up with a way to get out of some school work.

"He felt around my neck and said my glands were swollen," she said.

As she explained this to me, I flipped around on my back, practically yanking the phone cord out of the wall. I balanced the receiver under my chin and began to feel around my neck with both free hands. I felt two hard lumps on the right side of my neck. One of the lumps was right under my jaw bone, a good inch in front of my ear. The second mass was down farther, right above my collar bone. "My glands are swollen, too," I said, figuring that I, too, was probably coming down with a cold. "Hey, thanks for going to the dance and infecting me," I said.

Denial

Later that same evening, I stood in the shower, simultaneously flicking the knob on my yellow waterproof radio with my left hand and washing my neck with my right, pressing into my skin to better feel the lumps.

They were solid masses, each about the size of a quarter and the texture of a raspberry. While continuing to turn the radio dial in search of a good song, I made a mental note to tell my mom about the lumps. My mom always had an explanation for everything, and she knew how to fix what was wrong. This time would be no different, I figured.

That night, I mentioned the lumps to my mom. She felt them and guessed that it was some sort of drainage from a cold. Two weeks later, I had a routine physical with my pediatrician, and my mom mentioned the lumps. The pediatrician felt the lumps but, like both my mom and me, didn't appear to be too concerned. He had all kinds of theories about the origin of the enlarged lymph nodes. He supported my mom's cold theory and also suspected that it could be hormones or acne drainage. After all, these were typical preteenage problems, and I was a typical preteenage girl.

And then it happened.

"This is the age where we start seeing cancers common to the adolescent, but there is only a microscopic possibility that it could be cancer," the doctor said.

Looking back on it now, that one sentence changed my life. Hearing the word *cancer* made me cringe on a good day, but now the disease was being linked to me. When I heard the word *cancer,* I automatically thought of older people. Wasn't cancer a disease reserved for older people? I could recall my grandma telling my mom stories that proved it. My grandma would say something like, "It doesn't look good for Mr. Doomed. He is desperately sick." I knew "desperately sick" meant "cancer," and I knew that cancer was thought of as a death sentence. Could young people get cancer? Could young people die? My knotted stomach and sweaty palms hinted at the answers to these questions, but I couldn't comprehend the reality of it.

Rationalization

Still convinced that the lymph nodes were nothing serious, my mom and the pediatrician tried to calm my fears. The pediatrician referred my mom and me to a specialist at a local hospital to make sure that the lumps were harmless. I soon found myself under the care of an ear, nose, and throat doctor. This doctor ran blood tests and took chest x-rays, which came back with no evidence of cancer. The doctor concluded that it would be best to watch the swollen nodes to see if they would shrink on their own. The risk of performing a biopsy outweighed the risk that the swollen glands could be cancerous.

I was relieved. I thought to myself, This man is not only a doctor but a specialist, and if he says that I'm fine, then I'm fine. Plus, there is only a 1% chance that the lumps are cancerous.

Every day, I felt the swollen glands three times. They began to dictate my life. If the lumps felt particularly small that day, I had a good day and was confident that they would soon disappear all together. If the lumps felt bigger, I concluded it was probably because I had a cold or a sore throat caused by some persistent and undetectable allergy. Still, these types of days usually were bad days.

I put my life on hold twice a month to go back to the doctor so that he could do blood work and run chest x-rays and then tell me that everything looked fine. I kept telling myself, "If the tests are fine, you are fine." In reality, my doctor wasn't God. The test results were still in the normal range but indicative of high levels of increased white blood cell activity, and I wasn't fine.

Up to that point, the greatest tragedy in my life had been getting a B in freshman biology.

The summer of 1989 started out to be the best summer of my life. I had made it through my freshman year of high school, and for the first time in my life, I was holding down three baby-sitting jobs and enjoying having a steady source of income. I tried to ignore the swollen glands. In late June, I began to experience trouble breathing at night. At first, I tried to make myself believe that I was just developing severe allergies. After all, this could explain the whole enlarged gland riddle. Within three days, the whole right side of my neck was swollen, looking like it was about to give birth to a golf ball.

Shock

My mom and I went back to the doctor. When he saw my neck, his concern was unmistakable. He sent me to the radiology department to have a chest x-ray, and I just knew it was cancer—something that I had known deep down for two and a half years. My mom knew it, too. I could sense it, but she was trying to play it cool. Up until that moment, I don't think that I ever saw my mom as a real person. She was Mom, a virtual wonder woman, and I loved her, but she couldn't make this better. She and I both knew it. It was out of her hands. She was only human. This thought terrified me, and I can't imagine what it did to her.

I can still remember sitting in a dark, narrow hallway outside of the radiology department, waiting for the results of the chest x-ray. I cried. My hands felt like ice and my head ached.

An hour later, my mom, my doctor, and I were huddled together in a dimly lit room looking at my chest films illuminated against a white screen. That's when I saw it. It was a mass about the size of a grapefruit. It had waged war against my windpipe, causing it to deviate unnaturally from its poker-straight path. Unable to think or feel anything, I sat looking at the enemy for the first time. It was as if the real me was not in my body anymore and this experience was happening to someone who just looked like me.

Afraid that if he said it too loudly it would have to be true, a deflated doctor said in a small voice, "Katie, I'm sorry, but you have cancer."

In a few hours, my whole "old," secure, innocent, private world had become this new, unstable, uncertain, public world. In this new world, one question was answered that existed in the old world. Yes, young people do get cancer. Now, one question remained: Do young people die from cancer?

The rest of that day is still blurry in my memory. Mom and I went home with the knowledge that I was scheduled for an emergency biopsy the next day and that we had to induct others into our new world.

I remember crying all the way home and repeating over and over again, "I can't handle this."

Staging the Cancer

Uncertainty

The next two weeks were hell. The ear, nose, and throat doctor referred us to a pediatric hematologist/oncologist located at the same hospital. Several diagnostic tests were performed to determine the type and stage of my cancer. I thought it was never going to end. Being poked, probed, and prodded seemed unbearable. The tests were conducted on an outpatient basis, so I was able to go home after they were finished.

Each night when I finally got home, I went upstairs, straight to my room. I needed time to think, but I couldn't make sense out of anything anymore. Nothing was stable or certain, and this caused a level of anxiety that I had never experienced before—nor have I experienced since. It was as if I was falling down a seemingly endless well, knowing that when I hit the bottom, I was going to hit hard but not knowing when the impact was going to occur. One night, as I sat there on my bed staring blankly at my Strawberry Shortcake wallpaper, I remembered a mere 10 years back to when my parents finally gave in and let me have the wallpaper.

"You'll get sick of it in a few months," my father said. "But if you want it you've got it until you go off to college." Now I wondered if I'd ever make it to college, or through the summer, for that matter. Strawberry Shortcake might outlive me. In a desperate attempt to regain some control, I wanted to spring from my bed and start tearing the wallpaper down. I couldn't move. My body wasn't listening to me anymore.

About two weeks later, when all of the test results were in, it was time for the biggest test. I needed major surgery to biopsy all the lymph nodes in my immune system and my organs and to have my spleen removed. The surgery was scheduled for early the next morning, and I would be in the hospital for about two weeks. It was then, knowing what came next, that I hit the bottom of the well so hard that I broke through the ground and continued to fall.

A Brief Moment of Clarity

After the surgery, I knew what type of cancer I had and what stage I was in. The diagnosis: advanced Hodgkin's disease. In a sense, it was a relief. I took a deep breath and tried to imagine what was ahead of me. I couldn't. Fear of the unknown is a terrible thing. While questions were starting to be answered, so many unanswered ones still remained.

The Treatment

Trying to Accept the Situation

I remember sitting in a brightly lit hospital conference room with my oncologist and my parents. It was the day I was sprung from my two-week captivity/recuperation after the surgery. I felt a twinge of excitement—something that hadn't occurred in a long time, a feeling that I thought I had lost forever. But first we—my doctor, my parents, and I—had to decide on the course of my treatment.

Out of the corner of my left eye, I could see my chest x-ray again illuminated against a white screen. My mood darkened. There it was again, the enemy, ruining this good day. But, it was always there, I couldn't forget about it, and I didn't need an x-ray to remind me of it.

My doctor and parents were talking back and forth about treatment options as if I wasn't even there, as if it was about them and not me. I couldn't bring myself to say anything, but I wanted to say, "Excuse me, guys, but I'm right here. Don't talk about me like I'm not." At one point, my doctor suggested that I take a walk with one of the nurses. I knew they were going to start talking about death, and because it was *my* life and *my* death, I refused to leave.

Six cycles x four treatments per cycle = 24 chemotherapy treatments.

"Nationally, we have had the best results with this protocol, and Katie has an 80% chance of being cured using it. If you are going to get cancer, this one's a good one to get," my doctor said.

Somehow I tried to accept what she was saying. After all, she had a reputation for being one of the best in the oncology business. But the odds had been in my favor before and I had lost. I wondered, if this was a good cancer, what was a bad one like?

The First Chemo

I remember it like it was yesterday. I sit on the edge of a hospital bed, my arms extended in front of me. Two tightly tied tourniquets, secured right at the crook of each elbow, make any arm movement impossible. A chemotherapy nurse, strategically positioned between each arm, waits to pounce on any vein that dare raise itself to the surface of my pale skin.

In my mind, I plead, "Come on, will one of you guys just pop up already so I can get this over with?" I focus on my fingertips, which are beyond numb and wonder why my body has decided to mutiny on me once again. I've lost control of everything.

I can feel sweat beads trickling down my back, my eyes sting with tears that need to be cried, my arms ache from being kept for too long in an unnatural position, and my heart bangs against my chest as if it were a prisoner trying to make a last escape.

"So, are you right- or left-handed?" the nurse asks, with a sympathetic smile.

"Left. Why?" I say.

"The veins in the arm of the hand that a person uses to write with are exercised more and get more oxygen, so they are bigger and generally better at holding IV catheters."

"Oh," I say, shifting my gaze to my left arm. It seems like hours have passed and yet this process, the search for the proper vein to circulate my first-ever chemotherapy treatment throughout my entire body, has been going on for a mere 10 minutes.

"I got one," the nurse almost shouts as she plunges a needle into my right arm. I can feel it as it slices through my vein.

"Missed," she says.

Yeah, no kidding, I want to scream, but don't.

This whole "I got one/missed" thing goes on for another 10 minutes until the IV is finally secured in my right hand, but not before both of my arms and hands are lined with misses and I am lying down.

"You're a hard stick," the nurse says as she attaches a bag to my IV line and then mounts it on a pole.

There has got to be an easier way, I think to myself as I send an "I'm okay" smile over to my parents, who stand as close to me as they possibly can without being in the way of the nurse. They look scared. I don't ever remember them looking scared before.

The nurse attaches a blood pressure cuff just above the elbow of my left arm and then goes to get the doctor who will oversee my chemotherapy treatment. The cuff starts to inflate, and the pressure of it makes the needle sticks from the missed IV attempts sting. I can't believe this is happening.

I want to scream, "Mom, Dad, make them stop!" I want to rip out my IV and sprint down the hall and never come back; I want my doctor to burst into the room and say that she has made a terrible mistake and that I don't really have cancer; I want to be the 15-year-old girl I was a month ago—an innocent, ignorant child who thought she was immortal; I want to live, but I don't want chemotherapy, and if I don't have chemotherapy, I'll die.

Seconds later, a doctor appears. She is an older woman, in her early 60s. Her powdery white hair and tired, faded blue eyes seem to be road signs of a person who has seen too much, known too much. She reminds me of my grandmother. She explains that she is going to start my IV with Thorazine®. She says that Thorazine helps some patients with cancer because it combats nausea. I start to relax. Maybe I won't even get sick, I think to myself.

After the Thorazine, the doctor changes the bag on the pole. The new bag contains the first chemotherapy drug. I watch the clear contents of the bag slowly drip from the bag into my IV line and then into me. I start to feel sleepy, and when I swallow I notice a metallic taste in my mouth. A few minutes later, my head starts to throb and my whole body feels warm. I feel restless, and yet I can't make my body move. Three more drugs and an hour later, the infusion is over. The nurse and doctor help me to sit up, and I begin to feel dizzy. The doctor helps me to stand as the nurse gets a wheelchair. As soon as I stand, I feel my stomach start to contract, and before I can even sit in the wheelchair, I am overcome by six or seven dry heaves. My forehead erupts in sweat and feels so heavy that it takes extra energy to hold it up. When my stomach settles, I collapse into the wheelchair. I hear a voice in the background say, "Well, that's one treatment down."

My dad pushes me in the wheelchair while my mom races to get the car and pull it around to the front entrance of the hospital. I fade in and out of consciousness. I awaken in the car but don't remember how I got from the wheelchair to the car. The ride from the hospital to my house is about 20 minutes, and I know I'm not going to make it without getting sick. I get sick twice in the car, filling a "just-in-case bag" the nurse gave us for the ride home.

The next time I awaken I find that I'm on the family room couch. Every 10 minutes for six hours, I throw up. My stomach is sore, my nasal passages raw, and every time I prop myself up to throw up in the bowl at the side of the couch, my arms shake with tremors. I feel like I am going to die. And just when I think I'm not going to make it, like my stomach is going to burst, 10 minutes pass and I don't get sick. I start to get sick less and less until, finally, 10 hours later, I stop throwing up. And then I sleep for most of the next three days.

On the fourth day, I'm able to sit up and eat. And for the first time in my life, I truly enjoy feeling well.

Adaptation?

All totaled, my chemotherapy treatments lasted almost a year and a half. Those 15 months were filled with some extreme lows and some momentous highs, but what I remember most about that time were unique and often bizarre situations that arose because of my illness.

Because my immune system was weakened by chemotherapy treatments, before each visit to the orthodontist to have my braces tightened, I had to take penicillin to ward off any possible infections. I think my orthodontist thought that he'd kill me if he tightened my braces too tightly because every time he worked on my mouth, his hands shook violently and he'd constantly ask if he was hurting me. It's no wonder I had braces for seven years.

And then there were the times in my chemo cycle when I was taking a steroid called prednisone, a part of the chemotherapy regimen that is taken orally. This drug caused me to crave large quantities of one specific food for days and days. When I craved a certain food, I needed to have it. I went through Mexican, seafood, and Chinese phases. Prednisone also gave me insomnia. The weird thing was that my body would feel tired, but I had intense energy surges that I needed to act on. Often, in the middle of the night, I'd be wide awake and have more energy than I knew what to do with. And then there was the time, after my second chemotherapy treatment, that my doctor decided to surgically implant a catheter in a vein right under the surface of my skin to have easy access to my ever-disobedient veins. All of the nerve endings were cut around the area where the catheter, called a Mediport™, was placed. Now when a needle was put into the port, I didn't feel a thing and all of my blood work and chemotherapy could be administered through it. The only problem with my port was that sometimes it only worked when my body was in certain positions. One day, no positions were working. As a last resort, my doctor suggested that I do a headstand to aid gravity. Sure enough, it worked, and she was able to access the port while I was upside down.

Shingles

I had one more treatment left during the summer after my sophomore year in high school, and it looked like my junior year of high school would be normal. A week before school started, I noticed small, red bumps across my abdomen. At first, they itched, and then they started to sting—really sting. Each time I looked at my abdomen, the bumps spread further. Soon, I found myself sitting in my doctor's office. Shingles! Shingles sometimes occur in people who have a weakened immune system. Basically, once a person has chicken pox, the virus stays dormant in his or her body, and it can be reactivated when a person's immune system is compromised. Instead of getting chicken pox again, the person develops shingles along the course of nerves, which explains why this condition is so painful. I couldn't pass shingles on to anyone else, but I could give a person chicken pox if he or she never had it before.

My doctor admitted me to the hospital and started me on IV medications. I was beyond mad. I had been anticipating the start of my junior year all summer. Now I'd miss the first week, and to make matters worse, my final treatment was delayed.

I became so depressed and angry. I felt like I had come so far only to have a crushing setback. People visited and tried to cheer me up, but I wanted no part of it. I wanted to feel miserable.

After a week, I was released from the hospital. I was wiped out physically, mentally, and emotionally.

The Last Treatment

It's weird because I don't remember my last treatment. I waited and waited for the day to arrive, thinking that it never would. When the day finally came, it felt sort of unreal or too good to be true. I think that I got used to being sick. I felt safe in the sick world under the constant care of my oncologist. I never celebrated because I felt that I would jinx it and I would relapse.

What I do remember, vividly, was the first Thursday that I didn't have to go back for chemo. That was a great feeling.

On the Way Back Up?

At this point, I made an astonishing discovery about my whole cancer experience. It was harder to get back up than it was to fall in the first place. It's like that image of falling down the well, only now I had to climb back up.

Those first three months of remission were horrible. I was so tired physically. I couldn't even stand up long enough to take a shower, so I just sat down and let the water run over me. Getting a shower and getting dressed were my two big activities for the day. I also was mentally and emotionally exhausted. There were times during my treatment when I wouldn't let myself think about things or feel things. When my treatments ended, it all came back and hit me in the face. I spent those weeks in bed sleeping and crying and trying to make sense of everything that had happened. Slowly, I began to feel better. One day I was in bed, and I had this thought: Hey, stupid, you're alive! Why are you acting like you're dead?

At the beginning of November, I started back to school, and everything began to look a whole lot brighter. After a few weeks at school, I started noticing pain in my legs when I walked. I started to limp with my left leg. It hurt, but I thought it was because my muscles hadn't really been exercised for all these months.

One morning, I woke up and found that I couldn't walk at all. The next day, I was at the doctor's office.

The diagnosis: Avascular necrosis of the femoral head (AVN). I asked, "Is that cancer?"

"No," my doctor said.

That was all that mattered to me—it wasn't cancer. I thought it wasn't serious if it wasn't cancer. I was wrong.

I developed AVN in both of my hip joints because the prednisone I had received cut off blood flow to the tips of my hip joints, causing both joints to die and then collapse. Instead of having two rounded joints, I had two flattened hips.

I started going to see orthopedic doctors. The news wasn't very encouraging. Each one said something like, "We have never seen this condition in someone so young. You are going to need artificial hips."

To say that I became depressed would be an understatement. I felt like, "Come on, wasn't the cancer enough?" With each day, I was having more and more difficulty walking, and I was in constant pain. It hurt to do just about anything but lie down.

We did find one doctor who said that he could perform a procedure in which he would take my fibula and graft it into my hip joint to stabilize it and maybe get the blood flowing again. The surgery on my left hip was performed the summer before I started my senior year of high school, and I spent the first three months of my senior year being wheeled to class by friends. Surgery on my right leg was done the summer before I started college.

Today, I still have pain. Standing for long periods of time and walking great distances can be challenging. My left leg looks like it is about an inch shorter than the right, but actually they are the same size. The left leg looks shorter because the muscle is scrunched up. I have a lift in my left shoe, which isn't even noticeable. I know that hip replacement surgeries await me down the road. Sometimes I still get down about my legs and not being able to bend like other people, but the truth is that I have found ways to compensate. And sometimes people say stupid, insensitive things like, "Were you born with one leg shorter than the other?" The other day, a lady got into the elevator with me and asked, "What's wrong with your leg?" I turned and gave her a surprised look and said, "I don't know what's wrong with it." I also think about people who can't use their legs or have no legs. When it comes right down to it, I'd rather be alive and have hip problems than consider the alternative.

Back Up

I have been cancer-free for the last nine years. A few years ago, as I drove to meet my new adult oncologist at a new hospital, all of my old fears and anxieties began to resurface. My stomach started to knot, and my head was throbbing before I even parked the car. As I walked to the elevators, I felt weak. I had an urge to run away but couldn't.

I came alone this time. Having my parents there always seemed to make the situation more important, more serious. I wanted to prove to myself that I was a capable 23-year-old going for a routine, nonthreatening appointment, but when the nurse called me from the waiting room, I wanted my parents.

My appointment went well. As I sat in the waiting room expecting to be called to the laboratory for routine blood work, I noticed some bald, puffy-faced people—patients with cancer—who were waiting to undergo their treatments. I remembered myself, bald and puffy-faced, sitting in a similar waiting room. I remember wanting to be in remission, thinking it would never happen.

Surviving

I go through phases in which I rarely think about my cancer, and I go through phases where it is always on my mind. Sometimes, out of the clear blue and with no apparent impetus, I'll think, "My God, I had cancer, and I'm in remission." It's almost as if something, somewhere deep inside of me is trying to rationalize the experience. I went for my five-year checkup looking for some sort of promise, a guarantee. I wanted my specialist to tell me that my cancer would never come back because I felt that a guarantee would somehow finally erase my experience with cancer and liberate me by making all of my fears and anxieties about relapsing disappear.

But he couldn't give me a guarantee.

The absence of a guarantee has finally made me realize that even if all of the doctors in the world could promise that my cancer would never come back, I'd still worry that it would. I also realized that if I don't deal with my fears and anxieties, that even if I do not have cancer physically, I will be suffering from it.

Remission isn't just physical.

And yet, even though I possess this knowledge, there are still times when I am angry and scared and even terrified. However, while these times sometimes linger, they always pass.

When I was diagnosed with cancer, I thought I was going to die, but I thought wrong.

I once wrote a poem about my cancer experience, titled "The Aftermath." It deals with my feelings about letting go of my cancer experience and yet how it stays with me.

The Aftermath

They keep telling me it's gone
And I try very hard to believe.
They keep telling me it's gone
And after seven years of remission most would agree.
They keep telling me it's gone
But sometimes still nightmares come.
They keep telling me it's gone
Yet it has left me with a limp.
They keep telling me it's gone

Maybe, maybe there is not a single cancer cell?
They keep telling me it's gone
But would someone please inform the relentless voice in my head.
They keep telling me it's gone
But they didn't have Hodgkin's disease—I did!
They keep telling me it's gone
But what happens if it comes back?
They keep telling me it's gone
What they don't seem to understand is that for me, it can never be.
They keep telling me it's gone
And even though it is still with me, some days more than others, that's okay and I will go on.

Chapter 2.

Everything You Never Wanted to Know About Cancer

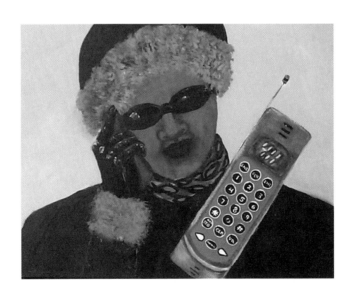

Chapter 2.

Everything You Never Wanted to Know About Cancer

Cancer 101—What Is It, Anyway?

Cancer is a generic term used to describe many different diseases, each with its own name and treatment. Cancer occurs when a cell or group of cells begins to multiply and grow out of control. Normal cells are then crowded out by these rapidly dividing abnormal cells, which are cancer cells (National Cancer Institute [NCI], 1993).

Following are some important facts that you need to realize about cancer (NCI, 1993).

Fact 1. Nothing you did or your mom or dad did caused you to get cancer. Cancer in younger people is unexplainable for the most part, and there is no evidence to suggest that you or those who love you could have done anything to prevent you from getting the disease.

Fact 2. Few cases of cancer in children and young adults are caused by genetics.

Fact 3. Your brothers and sisters are not more likely to get cancer because you have it.

Fact 4. Cancer is not contagious.

Fact 5. No food or food additive has been proven to be the cause of any childhood cancer.

Types of Cancer That Affect Teenagers

Leukemia

Leukemia is a cancer that occurs in the blood. It develops in the bone marrow, a sponge-like substance found inside your bone. The bone marrow is responsible for making blood cells (NCI, 1993).

The bone marrow makes three different kinds of cells. The red blood cells (RBCs) give the blood its red color. RBCs carry oxygen to the tissues inside your body. The second type of cells made by the bone marrow are known as platelets. Platelets help your blood to clot when you are injured and bleeding. The white blood cells (WBCs) are the last type of cells made by the bone marrow. There are three main kinds of WBCs. The neutrophils are responsible for destroying bacteria. The lymphocytes make the substances that are necessary to fight bacteria. The monocytes are important because they destroy foreign materials (NCI, 1993).

Leukemia involves the WBCs. When someone has leukemia, his or her WBCs are unable to mature. Instead of maturing, the cells remain young and immature and are not able to carry out their normal functions. Leukemia is not just one disease. There is a type of leukemia for each of the three types of WBCs. When a person has leukemia, only one kind of WBC is affected (NCI, 1993).

Leukemia also is classified as acute or chronic. When a person's leukemia is said to be acute, it means that it came on quickly and will keep moving rapidly without treatment. In chronic leukemia, the person's bone marrow is still able to produce some normal cells in addition to the cells that are leukemic. Chronic leukemia progresses more slowly than acute leukemia (NCI, 1993).

The diagnosis of leukemia requires blood tests and the examination of cells in the bone marrow (called a bone marrow biopsy). X-rays and spinal taps also can be used to determine if the leukemia has spread outside of the bone marrow.

When a person is diagnosed with acute leukemia, the type of WBC that has become leukemic needs to be identified.

The treatment for each type of leukemia is different. The type of leukemic cell involved usually can be determined by studying the cell under a microscope. Sometimes special tests of chromosomes and cell chemistry are needed to be absolutely certain of the type. Although very rare, sometimes the cells are too young and the type of cell affected cannot be identified. This type of leukemia is called acute stem cell leukemia or acute undifferentiated leukemia.

Leukemia may be treated by chemotherapy, radiation therapy, blood transfusions, antibiotic therapy, or, in rare cases, surgery (NCI, 1993). The goal of these treatments is to get the disease under control and destroy it. It may become necessary for a patient to undergo a bone marrow transplant if other treatments fail.

Solid Tumors

The word *tumor* does not always mean cancer. Some tumors, or collections of abnormally growing cells, are not cancerous. These tumors are classified as benign. A malignant tumor is a collection of abnormally growing cancer cells that has the capacity to invade and destroy normal tissue or spread to other parts of the body.

One type of solid tumor, known as sarcoma, affects the connective or supporting tissues, such as bone or muscle. Carcinomas are cancers that involve cells that line body tissues (NCI, 1993).

Lymphomas

Lymphomas are cancers that involve the lymphatic system. The lymphatic system is made up of vessels that carry lymph, an almost colorless body fluid, and the lymphoid organs, such as the lymph nodes, spleen, thymus, tonsils, and bone marrow. These organs produce and store infection-fighting cells. These cells are present everywhere in the body; therefore, lymphomas can develop in many different places (NCI, 1993). Lymphomas are divided into two categories—Hodgkin's and non-Hodgkin's lymphoma.

Hodgkin's lymphoma tends to involve lymph nodes near the surface of the body. Initially, the nodes in a specific area, such as the neck, underarm, or groin, start to swell. Hodgkin's lymphoma also is characterized by the appearance of a specific kind of cell known as the Reed-Sternberg cell (NCI, 1993).

An initial sign of non-Hodgkin's lymphoma may be swelling of the lymph nodes in the neck or abdomen. Additional symptoms of fever, weight loss, breathing difficulties, and problems swallowing may develop.

Lymphomas are diagnosed through a biopsy. A biopsy is a minor surgical procedure that involves taking a piece of the swollen lymph node and examining it under a microscope. The biopsy will determine if cancer cells are present and the type of tumor. Once the diagnosis is made, many tests are performed to determine the extent of the tumor. These tests can include bone marrow tests, computerized tomography (CT or CAT) and magnetic resonance imaging (MRI) scans, bone scans, and blood work. Treatment can involve radiation, chemotherapy, biologic therapy, or some combination of the three (NCI, 1993).

Brain Tumors

If a brain tumor is suspected, diagnostic tests such as skull x-rays, a brain scan, an MRI, or CT scans are done. Treatment depends upon the type of brain tumor. Often surgery, radiation, chemotherapy, or a combination are used. Recently, anticancer drugs that can penetrate the brain and central nervous system have been given intravenously or orally to treat brain tumors (NCI, 1993).

Neuroblastoma

Neuroblastoma occurs when very young nerve cells divide abnormally. Treatment options include surgery, radiation therapy, chemotherapy, or some combination of these treatments (NCI, 1993).

Wilms' Tumor

A Wilms' tumor starts in the cells of the kidney. Treatment options include surgery, radiation, chemotherapy, or some combination (NCI, 1993).

Rhabdomyosarcoma

Rhabdomyosarcoma or rhabdosarcoma is a soft-tissue sarcoma that involves the muscle cells. Treatment options include surgery, radiation, chemotherapy, or a combination (NCI, 1993).

Retinoblastoma

This is a relatively rare cancer of the eye and occurs in very young children. If it is diagnosed early, it is possible to destroy the tumor with radiation therapy and preserve normal vision. If the tumor is large and there is no hope of achieving adequate vision with radiation therapy, the eye is removed. In cases where both eyes are involved, an attempt is made to preserve vision in both eyes through radiation therapy. When advanced disease is found in both eyes, an attempt is made to preserve vision in at least one eye. If there is any possibility of useful vision, every effort is made to preserve it. Forms of treatment include chemotherapy, radiation, surgery, or a combination (NCI, 1993).

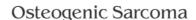

Osteogenic Sarcoma

Osteogenic sarcoma or osteosarcoma is a type of bone cancer that occurs in the ends of bones. The bones that are most frequently involved are the upper arm bone (humerus) or the bones in the leg (femur and tibia).

Although osteogenic sarcoma may be suspected by the way a bone looks, diagnosis only can be confirmed by a biopsy. The disease can spread to other parts of the body, such as the lungs. Treatment can involve amputation followed by chemotherapy. A prosthesis or artificial limb and physical rehabilitation are important to improve quality of life for these patients.

The use of implants and limb preservation is still in the experimental stages. In this process, the portion of the bone that is cancerous is removed and replaced with a special implant (NCI, 1993).

Ewing's Sarcoma

Ewing's sarcoma is different from osteogenic sarcoma because it affects a different bone. It affects the bone shaft rather than the ends of the bone. It tends to be found in bones other than the arms and legs—particularly bones such as the ribs. Treatment options include surgery, radiation therapy, chemotherapy, or a combination (NCI, 1993).

Common Diagnostic Procedures

Blood Work

Blood studies evaluate the components of the patient's blood and include the following.

- WBC count—The WBCs are those components of the blood that fight infection. Blood studies count the number of those cells per cubic millimeter (mm^3) of blood.
- Hemoglobin—This is the substance in the RBCs that carries oxygen to the tissues. Lower amounts than normal of hemoglobin indicate anemia.
- Hematocrit—The hematocrit is the percentage of blood that is made up of RBCs (Thompson, McFarland, Hirsch, & Tucker, 1993).
- Platelet—Platelets are the cells in the blood that help to stop bleeding.

CT Scans

CT scans are used for detecting masses in the body. During a CT scan, the person lies still on a table as a narrow x-ray beam, directed by a computer, revolves around the person's body. The beam travels through the portion of body being studied and the results are analyzed by a computer and appear as a three-dimensional image on a television screen. The image later will be developed into film.

Radioisotope Scans or Studies

Studies using radioisotopes are used to discover abnormalities in the liver, brain, bones, kidneys, and other organs. A harmless radioactive chemical is swallowed or injected, and the radioactive substance collects in the particular organ. Electronic devices are used to track the radioactive material as it collects within the body. By looking at how the material is distributed within the organ, the physician can see whether the organ is functioning properly or is abnormal.

Ultrasound Studies

Ultrasound studies use sound waves above the range of hearing that are bounced off tissue and changed electronically into images that can be examined. This procedure is helpful because tumors generate different echoes than normal tissue sound waves.

Bone Marrow Aspiration

This procedure helps to evaluate the cells that mature into normal blood cells. The procedure is usually performed on the hip bone. The patient lies on his or her stomach and the area where the needle is to be inserted is cleaned with an iodine solution to kill bacteria. The skin is then numbed with a local anesthetic. The needle is put through the skin and into the spongy part of the bone. Once the needle is in place, bone marrow is drawn into the syringe for analysis.

Biopsy

A biopsy is used to determine whether tumor tissue is benign or cancerous and to identify the type of the tumor. For this test, a small piece of tissue is removed from the tumor and examined under a microscope to check the cells. The tissue is examined by a pathologist, a doctor who is an expert at identifying changes in body tissue caused by disease. This microscopic study of tissue confirms or rules out a diagnosis of cancer and identifies the type of tumor cells that are present.

Lumbar Puncture

A lumbar puncture is used to determine whether cancer cells are present in the cerebrospinal fluid that surrounds the brain or spinal cord. It also can be used to directly administer drugs to the brain and spinal cord. The procedure is done while the patient is lying on his or her side and curled into a tight ball so that the lower back is rounded. A local anesthetic is applied to the lower back. The patient holds the position as the needle is inserted between the vertebrae into the fluid space around the spinal cord. A sample of fluid is withdrawn and examined for blood and cancer cells. Levels of sugar and protein also can be cultured to check for infection. After the fluids are collected, the patient may be given needed medications (NCI, 1993).

Cancer Treatments

Surgery

Depending on the type of cancer, a person who is diagnosed with cancer may have to undergo surgery for a variety of reasons. For the person with a suspected lymphoma, surgery will be used to take a biopsy so that an accurate diagnosis can be made. Surgery also will be used to determine the stage of the disease and to insert a port, the device used to draw blood and administer chemotherapy. Ask your doctor to explain everything about the need for a surgical procedure.

1. What does the surgery involve?
2. Will I be asleep for the procedure?
3. How will I feel when I wake up from surgery?
4. How long will I have to stay in the hospital?

Implantable Ports

Many different names can be used to describe these devices, and each one is a little different. A port is a piece of tubing that is surgically inserted into a vein. Chemotherapy and other drugs can be administered through the port, and blood work can be drawn through the port at the larger part of the tubing. The sensation of having an implanted port is that it feels like something the size of a quarter under your skin. The skin area around the port is numb because some nerves are cut during the surgery when it is implanted. The placement of a port saves a lot of vein poking and burning if it is inserted early in the course of your disease.

Chemotherapy

Chemotherapy is treatment with anticancer drugs. These drugs are administered in many different ways depending upon the type of cancer you have and how the drug or drugs should be administered. Drugs may be taken by mouth, injected into a muscle, given through a vein, or injected just below the skin. Another method used when treating brain tumors or preventing central nervous system disease in patients with leukemia is to inject the anticancer drugs into the spinal fluid (NCI, 1993).

Once in the bloodstream, chemotherapy drugs are absorbed by the rapidly dividing cells. In the cancer cell, the drugs interfere with the cell's ability to grow and multiply because they prevent the cell from dividing and deprive it of substances it needs to function. Eventually, the cell is destroyed (NCI, 1993).

Often, the bone marrow's ability to produce a normal amount of cells is affected. If the number of RBCs decreases, a patient may become anemic. If a person's platelet count becomes low, he or she may bruise or bleed more easily. When a person's WBC count is lowered, the person becomes more susceptible to infection (NCI, 1993).

Other side effects can include fatigue, nausea, vomiting, burning at the site of injection, hair loss, mouth sores, constipation, or diarrhea.

Radiation

Radiation therapy is treatment by high-energy x-rays. As the radiation interacts with cells, the DNA, or genetic code that directs development, is destroyed within the cells (NCI, 1993). The radiation doses kill the cancer cells but have a minimal effect on surrounding normal tissue. Side effects occur when the normal tissue is affected by the radiation and will depend on the area being treated.

The physician will mark the area that is going to be irradiated. The patient lies still while the treatment is being given, which just takes a few minutes. Areas of the body that are not being treated with radiation are shielded using lead aprons or shields. *You will not be "radioactive" or a danger to others if you receive external-beam radiation.*

Side effects of radiation therapy depend on the area of the body being treated and can include skin redness or irritation, sore mouth, hair loss, nausea, vomiting, diarrhea, and headaches.

Questions to Ask Your Doctor

Following are some questions that may be helpful when talking to your doctor about your cancer. It may be a good idea to write your doctor's answers down in a small notebook.

1. What kind of cancer do I have?
2. How is it spelled?
3. What part of my body does the cancer affect? Is it only in one place?
4. Can you recommend some books, booklets, or articles for me to read?
5. Do you know anyone that I can talk to who has had this kind of cancer?
6. What kind of treatment will I be having?
7. How does the treatment work? Do you have any information (booklets, films, or articles) on it?
8. If there will be side effects, what are they, how long will they last, and what can I do about them?
9. How often will I have to come to the hospital for treatment?
10. Can I keep going to school, or should I think about a home-based teacher? What about my activities?

Recurrence and Bone Marrow Transplants

Two issues that I haven't addressed in this chapter are recurrence, which is when a person's cancer comes back, and bone marrow transplant, a treatment that can be used for people who have received high doses of chemotherapy or radiation therapy that have damaged the bone marrow. The person will then receive an infusion of new cells to build the bone marrow (Cure for Lymphoma Foundation, 1998). Instead of giving a bunch of sterile facts, I thought it would be better to direct you to the personal accounts of those who have been through recurrence and bone marrow transplants. Andrea's story deals with both recurrence and a bone marrow transplant. Marc's and Bethany's stories deal with bone marrow transplants. Marc and Bethany both received marrow from people they didn't know who happened to match their bone marrow types, while Andrea received bone marrow from her sister. Their stories can be found in Chapter 8, "What Other Young Adult Cancer Survivors Have to Say."

This chapter was difficult for me to write because it involved many facts that I needed to research. I found the National Cancer Institute publication *Young People With Cancer* to be helpful. My goal was to gather as much information as I could about cancer in the teenager. I realize that this chapter doesn't account for all of the cancers that teens are diagnosed with; however, I hope it does give you a starting point or a frame for some of the terms or issues you are dealing with. The chapter "What Other Young Adult Cancer Survivors Have to Say" provides personal accounts of other young people who have dealt with many different types of cancer, procedures, and situations.

Cure for Lymphoma Foundation. (1998). Understanding non-Hodgkin's lymphoma: An introductory guide for patients. New York: Author.

National Cancer Institute. (1993). Young people with cancer: A handbook for parents (NIH Publication No.93-2378. Bethesda, MD: Author.

Thompson, J.M., McFarland, G.K., Hirsch, J.E., & Tucker, S.M. (1993). Diagnostic and laboratory studies. In J.M. Thompson, G.K. McFarland, J.E. Hirsch, & S.M. Tucker (Eds.), Mosby's clinical nursing (pp. 1371–1422). St. Louis: Mosby.

Chapter 3.

The Treaters

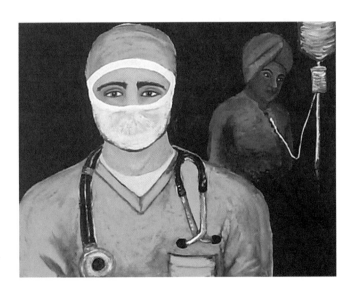

Chapter 3.

The Treaters

My new world, the hospital world, included new people who came to play very important roles in the treatment of my illness.

I knew how I felt about my illness (or at least there were brief, fleeting moments when I did), but I wanted to better understand the thoughts of people who, through their professions, deal with teenage cancer. As I talked to my pediatric social worker, a pediatric oncologist, and a psychologist in preparation for my book, I wished that I had sat down with my healthcare providers and asked these questions when I was going through my illness.

The first person I talked to was the pediatric social worker assigned to my case. During my treatment, I felt that she was the one person at the hospital on whom I could always count.

I met her the day I got my first bone marrow test. My parents weren't allowed to come into the procedure room with me. I had never thought about actually wanting my parents in the room with me until my doctor told me they couldn't come in. Then I wanted them there.

Once I got into the room, I started crying. Really crying. The social worker met me right inside the room. I didn't know who she was or what her role in this whole drama would be, but she became the person that I needed to be there. She introduced herself, and we started to talk about siblings and pets. I answered each question between sobs.

I don't even remember undressing and getting into that wonderful tie-on hospital gown. I just remember being on my stomach and waiting for the needle to go into my hip. She was sitting in a chair, positioned right in front of my face so that we had eye contact, and she was holding my hand. As the needle went in, she told me to take a deep breath, and as it came out, she told me to blow all of the air out. Although this seemed like a good suggestion, as soon as I felt the needle prick my skin, I starting screaming. By the time the procedure was repeated on my other hip, I was hoarse. No one had mentioned that they had to do the procedure twice, once in each hip, until they had me where they wanted me—with a nurse spread out over my back to keep me from moving.

After that test was over, I got up from the table and started to feel faint—and my backside was feeling more than a little sore. I couldn't believe I still had to go through more tests that day.

I now sat on a stool in the treatment room getting probed for another test by a very impatient intern, who was "jamming"—I mean trying to start—an IV in my hand. Suddenly, I broke out into a sweat and the voices around me started to sound very far off. I remember hearing the social worker say, "Do you feel okay?" The next thing I remember was awakening on the examination bed.

"I think I have had enough for today," I said.

"I think you're right," she said.

I got used to having her around. I liked her, and I especially liked talking to her. She even helped me to name my second cat. Ironically, we were having a conversation about pet names when I was undergoing a CAT scan. As usual, the needle was not going in well. We were bouncing names back and forth.

"How about Honey?" I said. "He's the color of honey."

"I don't know," she replied. "Does it fit his personality?"

"No, you're right. He's hyper," I responded.

The nurse interjected, "I just can't seem to find a vein. I'll try the other arm."

"You've got to be kidding," I scowled. "How many stupid tries do you need?"

"The more upset you get, the harder it's going to be to find a vein," she warned.

"I wasn't upset until you started digging into my veins."

"How about Chemo?"

"What?" I queried.

"You know, the cat. How about if you name him Chemo?"

"I don't think so."

"We are going to go ahead with the CAT scan even though we aren't going to be able to inject the contrast into your veins," the nurse informed me.

"What luck!" I replied.

The social worker commented on it being the luck of the Irish, to which I immediately responded, "Hey, what about Darby?"

"It's different. It's cute. It's Irish," she said. And that's how my cat came to be called Darby.

We lost touch after I finished undergoing treatment. As my treatments ended, she was moving to Chicago for a job opportunity. It took a few calls, but I was able to locate her. It turned out that she had moved back from Chicago and lived about 20 minutes from my house. As usual, we had a great conversation. It was so nice to be able to talk to her away from a hospital setting.

My first question to her was how a social worker fits into the picture for a teenager who is newly diagnosed with cancer. She explained, "Larger hospitals have social workers assigned to pediatric oncology floors. At smaller hospitals, a social worker could have several different assignments. At the hospital where you were treated, every new oncology patient meets with a social worker.

"A cancer diagnosis is a situation for which nobody is prepared. Social workers can help people in many different ways. They can direct people as to where to turn for answers to financial questions. For example, some organizations offer money to help patients to pay the cost of transportation to and from the hospital. Social workers also can help to facilitate communication. Often, a patient hears the word *cancer* and stops processing the rest of what's being said. If a patient has a question but doesn't want to ask or is afraid to ask, I'd say something like, 'This is what I'm hearing you say. Let me ask for you.' So I'm also there to go over information with patients.

"My role in relation to the medical team is to frame some of what is going on with the young adult and the family. Teenagers need to be in control, and there are ways for them to be able to keep control. For example, instead of someone saying, 'You are going to take your medicine now,' I'd step in and suggest the matter be handled by saying, 'You need to take your medicine. I understand that you might not want to take it now. I want you to take it by the time I come back.' A lot of time is wasted arguing.

"There is a perception that a patient needs a social worker because he or she is the problem, but it is the situation that is the problem. Here's where the emotional support comes in. You are not crazy; this is a crazy thing that is happening. I think it is important to give validation and tell people they have a right to feel horrible."

I next asked why she decided to become a social worker and work with kids and teens who have cancer. She explained that she actually was a theater major in college, although during her senior year, she realized that other students were getting better parts than she was. After graduating from college, she taught a theater class for a program called Upward Bound, a college prep program for kids with problems. "Kids just started coming to me and telling me their problems," she explained. "They seemed to feel better after we talked. I began to feel strongly about my role in making the world a better place and decided to go into social work." At that point, she had only taken one psychology class and no sociology classes, so while working in a library for two years, she began to take classes such as adolescent psychology, with the intention of going into child welfare—she knew nothing about pediatric oncology.

She further explained, "One day while at work, a doctor asked me to help a newly diagnosed patient with cancer in dealing with a spinal tap and a bone marrow test. As I walked into the treatment room, all of the doctors were there, ready to perform the procedure. I walked in with my puppet, Rozzi, on my hand. Rozzi is a furry raccoon hand puppet with its own hospital name tag. Everyone looked. When I saw the two procedures being done, I nearly fainted. It was interesting to me because after each procedure was done, the boy wanted to look and see the fluids that had been taken out of his body. I think this is a way for patients to stay in control and prove that they went through this for a purpose." As she said this, I smiled because I had asked to see my bone marrow after the test. It really did look neat. It was red from the blood and sort of spongy-like.

The social worker believes that being a theater major helped her with being a social worker. As she explained, "An actress feels the feelings of a character but expresses those feelings in a way that relates to the audience. She is always conscious of her props. An actress has to be aware of her verbal and nonverbal movements as well as others' verbal and nonverbal communication. Active listening is a must. I feel this when I am with a family and bad things happen. I have to be aware of how I relate so that I do so in a way that will help the family. Sometimes I will cry, but I must remember that the family shouldn't be comforting me. This is very similar to what being on stage is like."

I next proceeded to explain that for a long time I was very hostile toward people who didn't have cancer because I felt that they couldn't possibly know what it was like.

I resented having to go and talk to a shrink who had never had cancer but was supposed to help me deal with cancer. I asked how she would respond if someone told her that she couldn't possibly know what it is like to have cancer. Again, she returned to her theater training in her response. She said, "I'd say you're right, I don't know what it is like to have cancer. I also don't need to be a murderer to play the part of a murderer. I have been educated in the effects of illness. I also have learned through experience that control is a huge issue for teens who are undergoing treatment for cancer. I studied child development, and I can imagine what it would be like for me. But I can only imagine. I think the key is to listen. A real awareness of another's feelings can be achieved. It is like playing a character that is so totally different from my personality. I find something in that character that I can relate to. With my patients, it's about finding a way to connect with them."

I asked her to share her advice for teens being treated for cancer. "I would tell them that it is okay to have awful feelings," she replied. "It is important to find ways to express anger. Setting short-term goals is a good way to gain back some control. You should be proud of yourself. You are doing something very hard. Don't think you always have to be brave. Find your source of strength."

She also described some of the major issues she has seen in working with teens over the years. Control is the main issue. "Teens are engaged in a struggle between independence and dependence," she explained. "Cancer throws teens back to a more dependent time. Many foundations are shaken. For example, this whole sense of invincibility and immortality is taken away. There is isolation from peers who are tired of hearing about it, can't relate, and don't want to deal. There are appearance issues. There are interruptions to a teen's life in every realm. There are sexuality issues, such as, 'Am I going to be able to have children?'"

For me, the social worker was the key in my treatment plan. She was the one I wanted there. She kept me company during procedures in which my parents weren't allowed to be present. My doctor always walked in the room and said, "I paged her. She'll be here in a minute."

I had several questions that I felt I needed to ask a pediatric oncologist. I didn't think I'd be able to go back to the hospital at which I was treated, nor did I think that I'd be able to talk to my adult oncologist about teenage cancer. I can't even go into the hospital where I was treated without becoming violently ill, and I didn't want to face my pediatric oncologist because I was embarrassed about how I acted at different times during my treatment. I took the safe road and found another pediatric oncologist to talk to.

While I sat and waited to talk to the pediatric oncologist, I noticed a little girl and her parents and brother sitting in the waiting room. I overheard the mother talking to the receptionist and heard that the little girl had leukemia. She was newly diagnosed. I felt the tears in my eyes. I watched as the mother and child walked over and joined the dad and brother at the opposite end of the waiting room. The little girl was crying because she didn't want to get an IV today.

I thought to myself, How many three-year-olds know about IVs?

A few minutes later, I was called back into the doctor's office. I liked him as soon as I met him. I could feel how much he cared about kids and teens with cancer.

Our conversation went easily. I first asked him to define in his own words what cancer is. "When I tell a teenager that he or she has cancer, he or she pretty much knows what it is and the implications of it," he responded. "When I am giving a family a diagnosis, I always talk to the patient and the parents. I talk about the therapy and how we will be treating the cancer. I then ask the child or teen who has been diagnosed, 'What does cancer mean to you?' I feel this is an issue that needs to be addressed right away because it really breaks down barriers. I often see parents protecting their child and the child protecting his or her parents."

"What advice do you offer?" I asked.

"I'm always realistic and hopeful," he said.

"No matter what?"

"Yes."

I asked the oncologist how much the teen's input is taken into consideration.

"They are always included," he said. "Teens really do have more control than they first realize. Examples of issues in which teens have control include, but are not limited to, standard treatment protocol versus clinical trial (which is a treatment protocol that is still being evaluated) and if they want to get a central line for administration of chemotherapy and what type of line to get. They also have choices about being admitted to the hospital. The patients do have control within reason."

I next asked, "If there was one crucial thing that you'd want a teen undergoing cancer treatment to know, what would it be?"

He replied, "We are going to do everything we can to fight this. Different patients pick up on different aspects of their illness at different times. I gear the fight to what a patient picks up on. I tell each patient what is necessary, and then I wait and listen. The hard questions usually come later."

Finally, I asked why he had decided to become a pediatric oncologist. He said, "There is an overwhelming need for consistent compassion in this field. I see families in the worst circumstances, and yet I'm impressed with how they deal with cancer and go on with life. The transformation from a sick child to a healthy child is an amazing process filled with many ups and downs, but it is worth it when I see a child fighting and growing healthier and stronger."

Even though I had this wonderful conversation with a pediatric oncologist, I still felt that it was necessary for me to speak with my own pediatric oncologist. I needed some closure. I transferred to an adult oncologist when I turned 20 and haven't been to the hospital or seen her since. Part of me was still angry about some of the things that had happened during my treatment—things that were easy to blame on my doctor that were in no way her fault. Much of my anger was directed at her during the duration of my treatment. In my mind, she was the one making me sick and imposing all of those restrictions on me when, in actuality, she was the one who saved my life.

I felt I needed to apologize. I felt I needed to say, "Thanks for saving my life."

A few weeks later, I was looking for a parking space in the hospital's garage. As I entered the building, I smelled that smell. It all just came back to me, and I ran to the nearest bathroom. Leaning over the toilet, I vomited like I used to after chemotherapy.

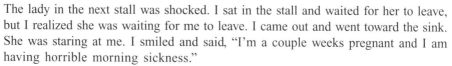

The lady in the next stall was shocked. I sat in the stall and waited for her to leave, but I realized she was waiting for me to leave. I came out and went toward the sink. She was staring at me. I smiled and said, "I'm a couple weeks pregnant and I am having horrible morning sickness."

"Oh," she said and smiled.

I felt so much better after that, and by the time I met my doctor, I was feeling probably the best I've ever felt at that hospital. Upon meeting, we caught up on each other's lives and families.

I began by asking her, "How would you respond to the patient blaming himself or herself and saying that he or she caused the cancer? Likewise, how would you respond to the family who is blaming themselves?" She said that she would emphasize that neither the patient nor the family in any way caused the cancer.

I next asked her to identify the single most important thing that she wants a recently diagnosed teen to know and what advice she would offer for the recently diagnosed teen and family.

"Usually as soon as people hear that they have cancer, they tune out," she explained. "I give statistics on the cure rate. I feel that the more information that is given to the patient, the better the trust and honesty. I always meet with the family and the patient again shortly after they are given all of this overwhelming information. I encourage them to write their questions down, and I tell them that I will answer these questions and explain the information again until they understand. I also can offer other supports, such as social work and the child life department. The child life department deals with children's needs in relation to hospital encounters; however, they are more oriented to smaller children and not teens."

Last, I asked why she decided to become a pediatric oncologist. She answered, "When I was growing up, my sister, who is 10 years younger than I am, was very sick. I know what it is like for families who are dealing with chronic disease and are in chaos. I wanted to help others."

My pediatric oncologist told me that she totally understood why I had acted the way I had.

At one point in my treatment, I was referred to a psychiatrist by my oncologist. I was angry about this and didn't give him a chance. I felt like I had every right to lose my mind. Now, when I look back, I think that talking with someone in the mental-health profession about what I was going through would have been helpful. I found the psychologist's comments to be so true to what I had experienced when I was sick that I felt like he was reading my mind.

I didn't know this psychologist while I was going through treatment. He focuses on treating anxiety disorders and anxiety reduction. I asked him about the issues that he felt were especially relevant for teens with cancer, and he said that communication issues are huge for teenagers. He explained that teenagers who are diagnosed with cancer often feel as if they are defective.

"I work with teenagers on desensitization," he said. "I want them to be more comfortable with themselves and with their illness. We also do role playing and work on ways to educate others about their illness."

The psychologist also talked about compliance being another big issue. "We work on reexamining the doctor-patient relationship," he said. "This includes, but is not limited to, issues such as assertiveness." He explained to me what happens when he first meets with a patient. "I always tell the patient that he or she doesn't need to be here. I meet with the teen for half an hour. Then I meet with the parents for half an hour. Then we meet together."

Personally, I was curious about the issues that arise because of cancer and still exist after the person goes into remission. I explained that I spend much time thinking about the role that cancer still plays in my life. I don't think this is good or bad; it's as if I'm just trying to make sense of it all.

He said, "Instead of asking, 'Why me?' why not ask, 'What do I want to create?' It's really not about fixing something that is wrong or was wrong but creating reality."

What do I want to create?

Chapter 4.

Hair: It Really Does Grow Back

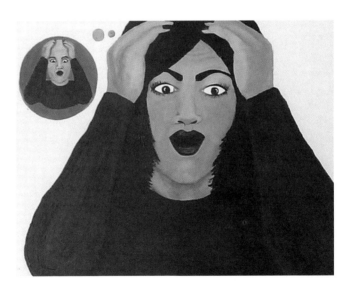

Chapter 4.

Hair: It Really Does Grow Back

People Undergoing Chemotherapy Often Experience Hair Loss

When chemotherapy drugs get into the bloodstream, they affect rapidly dividing cells. If the cell is cancerous, the drugs stunt the cell's attempts to divide and grow. Anticancer drugs cannot determine which cells are good and which are bad. These drugs target all cells that grow and divide rapidly. Hair cells grow rapidly. The drugs destroy rapidly dividing cells such as hair cells resulting in hair loss.

People Undergoing Radiation Often Experience Hair Loss

Radiation therapy involves treating cancer with powerful x-rays. High levels of radiation can kill cells or keep them from growing and dividing. As previously mentioned, cancer cells grow and divide quickly, as do hair cells. Hair often is lost in the area receiving radiation.

Important Facts to Remember

1. Hair loss is a reversible side effect that will generally improve after the chemotherapy or radiation is stopped.
2. Hair loss may even stop while a patient is still receiving active treatment.
3. If you lose less hair than someone else who also is in treatment, this does not mean that your treatment is less effective.

Strategies for Coping With Hair Loss: Physical

Wigs

I wore a wig to school and to other social functions. A good wig probably is the best way to look as much like the before-cancer-you (BCY) as possible, the key words being "a good wig." I often hear about people getting wigs and wearing them only occasionally. I must admit I was glad to have it, but after a while I began to wear it less and less.

Wigs do have their drawbacks. They can be hot in the summer, a major pain to securely fasten when going certain places (such as amusements parks), and a potentially life-threatening hazard to cats, who for some bizarre reason are attracted to them like they are to catnip. We are talking major hairball here!

Hats

I wore a hat in the summer and in situations where I was comfortable with the people around me. Hats are cooler, allow for many color and style change options, and can be color-coordinated with socks and other accessories.

On the down side, people might stare at you when you are wearing a hat. Several times, I was mistaken for a boy. Hats also tend to fall off more easily than wigs.

Scarves and Turbans

Scarves and turbans are nice to wear either under a hat or by themselves. They are even cooler than hats and can be wrapped in very elegant ways around the head. I rarely wore these, but when I did, I usually wore big, floral print ones so that everyone knew I was a girl.

Au Naturel

The only time that I went around without anything covering my bald head was when I was at home. Even then, I kept a hat or scarf nearby in case someone rang the doorbell. This option will leave you coolest in hot weather and the coldest in winter. If you choose this option, people probably are going to stare at you or perhaps even make some comment. I think it's a good idea to arm yourself with some good comebacks so that you can head off the pondered or spoken question, "What happened to your hair?"

My all-time favorite response to that question is, "I don't know, what happened to it?" This is probably going to sound mean, but I like that response because it catches the person off guard and shifts the uncomfortable feelings of the situation to the person who asked the question.

I realize that this is a somewhat biased account of what to do when you are losing your hair. Several of my male friends, who have written stories in Chapter 8, "What Other Young Adult Cancer Survivors Have to Say," informed me that they either wore a hat or went au naturel.

Strategies for Coping With Hair Loss: Emotional

The only way I know how to help you emotionally is by telling you how I felt and what I experienced. When I lost my hair, I was devastated, but not as devastated as I thought I would be. The one thing about cancer is that it sets your priorities straight. If I had been a normal teenager and then one day woke up with all of my hair gone, I think I would have died. But when cancer entered the picture, hair loss was just one more of the temporary battles in a much larger war.

I began to realize that when it came down to my hair or my life, my hair could be replaced. It was one of those realizations that often was tempered by depression, sadness, anger, jealousy, rage, and pity, and yet in the midst of all of these emotions, I knew it to be true. My bald head set me apart from people, especially my peers. I was different in a society that advocates conformity. Sometimes people stared; sometimes I stared back and sometimes I didn't. Sometimes when people talked to me, they couldn't even look me in the eye because all they could see was the wig or the hat or the scarf. Sometimes I made it so they had to look at me, but sometimes I was too sick and too tired to care. Sometimes I bit my lip in anger when my friends talked about their bad hair days. At least they were able to have them. Sometimes I held back hot, jealous tears when my peers talked about the latest hair styles and experimented with the latest trends. Sometimes I longed for hair so badly that I brushed other people's hair and pretended it was my own; every time, I reminded myself that my hair would grow back.

What I Learned in Dealing With My Own Hair Loss

A person who is undergoing treatment for cancer has to remember that, in most cases, his or her hair is going to grow back. This is not a permanent situation. I always kept this thought in the back of my mind. While the loss of my hair was devastating, I survived it. Hair is not necessary to sustain life.

Cancer treatments not only destroy the bad cells but also the good ones, and because hair is nourished by the good cells and it is being destroyed, it only follows that the bad cells are getting decimated as well.

I am still the same person—hair or no hair.

What Someone Else Taught Me About Hair Loss

Eight years ago, I didn't know what to expect when I walked into a hair replacement and cosmetic center. Deep inside, I was feeling painfully self-conscious because my hair was starting to fall out and I needed to do something about it. Outwardly, I was furious because I didn't want to have to be there. I had enough of cancer and all of its ugly side effects. I thought that getting fitted for a wig was going to be one of the most embarrassing and humiliating experiences of my life. I was wrong.

My anger started to dissolve as soon as I walked into the salon. The lobby was warm and inviting, lined with awards and plaques from all over the world that the owner had won for his work in training and certifying cosmetic therapy centers specifically designed for helping patients with cancer.

And then I saw something that just made me smile: a testament to the importance of the owner's work by one of his youngest clients.

It was a picture drawn in crayon that is framed and placed in the center of the lobby, an illustrated mission statement of sorts. The picture is divided into two squares. In the first square, there is a picture of a bald, frowning child. Slightly above the child's head is a large cloud that completely blocks the sun. In the second square, the child, complete with a new wig, is smiling and the sun shines high above the child's head. Before I even met the owner, I knew I was going to like him. I was right. When I shook his hand, I felt immediately at ease. He was then and is now more like an old friend. Somehow he just knew me and knew how I felt about losing my hair.

On that first visit, he took a sample of my hair and we talked about how I wanted my wig styled. A few weeks later, I had my wig, and I had to admit that it would do.

I often came back to the salon during my year and a half of chemotherapy for cuts and style changes. We even sat for hours and managed to work my wig into a French twist for my sophomore dance.

Many months later, we rejoiced together when my real hair was long enough to be cut and styled again.

A Hair-Raising Experience

The first summer that I was sick, I decided to go to a local amusement park with my friend and her youth group. As the day of the outing got closer and closer, I became more worried. I had these nightmares about my wig flying off on the highest hill of a roller coaster right onto the track. The roller coaster runs over it, and the wig gets caught in the wheels, causing the roller coaster to veer off the track. Everyone is killed except me. I survive cancer but get sued for the rest of my life.

Looking back, I should have said, "The heck with it all" and just worn a hat or painted my bald head with some saying like, "Queen of all roller coasters." However, I remember how anxious I was about this and soon found myself calling the cosmetologist for advice. A few days later, I stopped by his office to pick up some industrial-strength wig glue. He warned me to read the directions carefully. So I went home and read the directions. In bold print it said, "Apply at least an inch away from hairline. Do not get in hairline." I dismissed the directions, excited and relieved that I wouldn't have to worry about losing my wig the following day.

The next morning, I applied the glue to my wig. My wig didn't seem secure enough so I put some glue on my finger tip and shoved it up into my wig. Then I was off.

I think I rode every roller coaster at the park and had no problems with my wig staying on. In fact, it didn't move once. Later that evening, I came home and began to get ready for bed. I soon found that my wig was stuck to my head. I tried pulling it gently, but I immediately felt little hairs tearing. "Oh God, I got the glue in my hairline." Well, I couldn't get the wig off. I was beginning to think that I was going to have to cut it off.

I called my mom upstairs, and for the next few hours we gently worked at detaching it from my head. I was in pain. We used nail polish remover. My head was soaked with sweat and nail polish remover. In order to get the final piece of my head free from the wig, my mom and I really had to pull. It felt as though a piece of my scalp was being pulled off. Sure enough, along with the wig came a rather significant portion of my scalp. When I looked into the mirror, I had a bloodied bald spot about the shape of a raisin. To this day, I still have that bald spot.

A Final Thought

Take comfort and know that soon you'll be sprouting this soft, fuzzy, baby-fine hair. But beware. People soon will take liberties to rub your head whenever they feel like it and say things like, "Oh, how cute," or "It's so soft." And as the after-cancer-you, the ACY, embarks on your second "first haircut," know that it is one of the best feelings in the world.

Chapter 5.

Relating

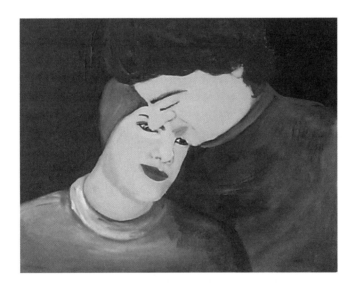

Chapter 5.

Relating

Cancer touches everyone who is connected with the person who has it. I knew how it felt to have cancer, but I didn't know how it felt to be a parent whose child has cancer, a sibling of a person with cancer, a friend of someone who has cancer, or a significant other of someone who has cancer.

Many of the stories in Chapter 8, "What Other Young Adult Cancer Survivors Have to Say," explore how parents, siblings, friends, and significant others coped with their loved ones' diagnoses as seen through the eyes of the person being treated for cancer.

A big part of relating to someone is trying to see where he or she is coming from. So, here are some thoughts from parents and siblings who have been touched by cancer.

Melba M. Valarezo, the mother of Maria Valarezo, whose story appears in Chapter 8, shared three poems she wrote as her daughter battled leukemia.

A Mother's Helplessness

Begging for the nightmare to end;
While knowing it just begins;
Her mind is numbed by the pain;
Tears run openly without shame;
Sitting watch by her sick child's bed;
Mother's helplessness is felt in depth;
A scream from within almost chokes;
Escapes as a whimper from her throat;
She prays for God to heal;
"Please, let it be Your will."

Healing of Maria

God, thank you for saving the life of this daughter of mine;
For giving her strength during fearful times.

Your nearness to her side keeps her spirits high;
In the midst of pain, she responds with only a sigh.
Father, in Your wisdom, You know well the truth;
Earth needs her here more than heaven and You do.
We all enjoy the compassion and humor she freely gives;
We're grateful for her healing, letting her live.

Hope

Hope dwells within the heart of man,
Sparking the fires of "Yes, I can!"
Its very essence fuels our dreams,
Motivating them into realities;
Hope lightens the darkest halls of fear,
Allowing focus upon brighter times near;
Hope brings out the best man can be,
A wonderful spirit fulfilling dreams.

Musings of a Mother of a Child Who Has Survived Teenage Cancer

By Karen Gill (my mom)

Things I learned:

- That I had the quiet support of friends
- To laugh at quirky things—like the doctor who looked as if he had just stepped off the set of "Mr. Roger's Neighborhood"
- A new perspective
- That you can get through anything life throws at you
- To be more forgiving of human frailty
- That when I was sure God had given me about all I could handle, there was still more He asked
- That hospital chairs are not conducive to sleep; that the human body is not meant to rest in the vertical position
- That hospital rooms are too small
- That doctors should practice being patients
- That it's difficult to quiet the panic in someone else when your own heart is thundering in your ears
- To despise comments like "I know exactly how you feel," "It could be worse," or "If you're going to get cancer, this is the best kind to get!"
- Not to say those things to others
- To come to terms with the fact that people just don't know what to say to you
- To hate emesis basins
- To hate the night before chemo and the days after

- To be so possessive that I didn't want to share my daughter with anyone
- To let go
- That a depressed immune system and shingles don't mix
- That there are many beautiful, caring people in the world
- That wigs just don't cut it
- To hate stares
- In order to have something—life—you have to give something up
- That scars are beautiful
- Yes, indeed, I can flush a Mediport™
- That cats are not supposed to invade a sterile field
- That the rough, tough times that came before were there for a reason; they were only practice runs for the main event; God was getting me ready, but I didn't know it
- A lot about guilt, the "If only, what if, why her, why me, why not me, why them, why?"
- To cry, unabashedly and unashamedly
- That good things do, indeed, come out of bad
- To be more open to people and their problems, realizing that you have no idea of the pain they are dealing with
- To prioritize
- That there will always be jerks, or rather "people who are becoming"
- That the journey up takes so much longer than the ride down

My Sister Chose Life

Melba Joelin Valarezo shared the following essay she wrote about her older sister, Maria.

Walking to the bus and expecting my sister to be there riding home with me, I remembered being unsure of whether she would die or be there for the events we had always talked about—graduations and weddings. Remembering how it feels to be afraid of losing her to cancer reminds me to not take things for granted. Remembering is like walking down a long hospital hallway, looking in the room, and making sure she is still there and hasn't faded away into the white hospital sheets.

It seemed like any other day at home after school, but this day we'd always remember, for it is embedded in our minds with tears. Day turned to night after one fateful blood test set the roller coaster going full speed. The destination was unknown. Thinking of it as any other sickness, I came home to visit with my sister, eager to tell her about my day. After receiving a phone call, I felt slapped by an intense, tearful silence that sent us packing to the hospital. Packing for the trip, we let tears slip like raindrops down our cheeks for each nameless fear we were to face. After reaching the hospital, I had to leave her behind to go back home to find an empty room suspended in time. I asked my mom what was wrong. Stuttering and sick, my mom answered my question with one word—leukemia. She told me that there was a possibility that my sister, Maria, had it.

I watched helplessly as my sister aged before my eyes with chemotherapy, radiation therapy, spinal taps, and bone marrow tests. It seemed like she would never see the end of so many needles. She aged emotionally through sadness, pain, and courage. Setbacks built upon setbacks, but Maria would just laugh it off, letting tears out through her laughter. A two-month side effect caused two months that seemed to last forever, cut off her music, her laughter. Maria could not be treated for two months, which resulted in depression. It crushed our hearts, seeing her free-fall without her net, her family. Finally, one of us woke her out of her seemingly endless trance of depression. Maria was back.

Days, weeks, months, years passed us in a blur. Sudden shock, pain, and sorrow left us wiser, but with many memories and tears. My sister almost gave up many times, but she chose life. Laughing, playing games, or just talking with her, I feel overwhelmed with happiness just to have her here with us. Without Maria, there would be such a big hole in our hearts.

My sister tells me it was hard; she wouldn't wish it on anybody else, but she wouldn't take it back. My views and definition of cancer have changed because of my sister. I used to associate cancer with death. I now associate it with hope, support, faith, and surviving.

It sounds ironic, but when it was happening, I was brave and strong, acting as a rock for my sister to lean on. Now it seems that just remembering the experience brings tears to my eyes. I guess now is my time to cry for my sister and all of the other patients with cancer. Maybe, just maybe, I cry for the little girl who saw her sister grow weaker and weaker.

A Song to My Brother

I met the Buckley family through a local hospital. I soon found myself being warmly welcomed into their house. Marshall Buckley, a 15-year-old survivor of Hodgkin's disease, his younger brother, Matthew, their parents, and I looked back on our often similar cancer experiences while enjoying dinner.

Mrs. Buckley shared a song that Matthew had written for Marshall. As I read it, my eyes started to sting with tears. After I finished, I asked Matt if I could include it in my book. He said, "Sure!"

The song starts with a dedication:
To my brother, Marshall. Love ya. Matt

Live Awhile

If you're going to fly,
Please don't fly away.
If you're going to die,
Please don't die on me.
So hold on.
Can't you see I love ya so,
And I know you love me, too.
So, hold on, please don't die on me.
Please just try to live awhile, to live awhile.

Can't you see I love ya so,
And I know you love me, too.
'Cause me and God know you're strong,
Can't you see I need ya,
So please don't leave me to stay down here.
Can't you see I love ya so,
And I know you love me, too.
So please just live awhile, live awhile,
Live awhile,
Please just live awhile.

I Remember

I feel that the another important part of this chapter is how people with cancer relate to their parents, brothers and sisters, friends, and significant others.

I remember after I was first diagnosed, I tried to make my parents get mad at me. I wanted them to treat me like they did before I got cancer.

I remember after I was first diagnosed, I was getting a steady stream of cards, gifts, and flowers. It was so touching, and I appreciated the thoughtful gestures from friends, family, and even people I didn't know. One day, just after another package had arrived, my younger brother said, "You're so lucky to be getting all this stuff." My dad then said, "I'm sure she'd give it all back to be healthy again."

I remember my older brother getting mad at me and yelling, "You know, you're not the only one with problems."

I remember calling one of my friends to tell her that I had cancer and her saying, "Oh, don't worry. You'll be fine. Well, I've got to go now."

I remember being at a dance and becoming totally overwhelmed by how hot it was inside the gym and feeling like I was going to pass out. My date had no idea what to do.

But I Also Remember...

I remember both of my parents always being there for me.

I remember my younger brother coming to visit me at the hospital and bringing a box of candy and a Slinky®. There were tears in his eyes.

I remember my older brother telling me that the best news he ever heard was when I told him I was in remission.

I remember my friends writing cards for me in school and bringing them over.

I remember my date for the junior prom bringing me carnations and sitting with me because I was too sick to go to the dance.

There were times when I felt misunderstood by my friends and my family. There also were many times when I made it hard for my family and friends to understand me.

For every time that I felt I was mistreated by someone who "claimed" to love me, there was another time when that person showed me such great love that I felt ashamed for ever being upset with that person in the first place.

The most important advice I feel that I can give to anyone with cancer about relating to parents, siblings, friends, and significant others is to tell them how you are feeling. I think that sometimes I expected people to read my mind. In addition, I know this is easier said than felt, but people who are your real friends will stick by you. If they don't, they weren't worth having as friends in the first place.

Chapter 6.

The "Why" Questions

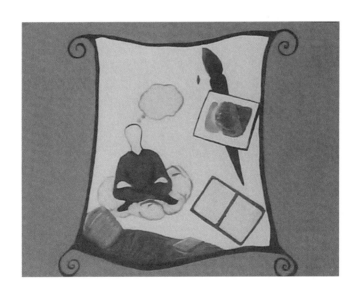

Chapter 6.
The "Why" Questions

Why Me?

For me, and maybe for you, as well, these questions seem to have a religious slant. In no way do I want anything in this chapter, or anywhere else in this book, to sound like I am preaching. I hate being preached to, and I would never do it to anybody else. This is simply my explanation of how I have dealt with what I call the "Why" questions and how I tried to seek answers.

While I was raised Roman Catholic, this chapter is not a Catholic explanation of suffering. I'm not even sure what a Catholic interpretation of suffering would be, or if there is such a thing. It is very simply me trying to find answers to questions, knowing that I might never be satisfied with what I found or continue to find. For a long time, my cancer diagnosis seemed to bring more questions than answers. The very first question, "Am I going to die?" always was in the back of my mind, and new questions always were forming. "Why me?" "Why am I being punished?" At this point, the whole shock of learning that I had cancer was starting to wear off, and I was becoming angry.

Actually, this is a major understatement.

At times, I was so angry that my body convulsed with spasms. I cried hot, angry tears but only ended up with puffy eyes, flushed checks, and a splitting headache. My rational self then thought, "Oh, great, now I have a brain tumor." It couldn't be just a headache, I thought. I screamed and swore and threw objects, breaking a few. I was surprised and scared at the intensity of my anger; there were times when I really thought I was going to explode like a bomb and shatter into a million pieces.

The hours right before I was to receive a chemotherapy treatment always were the worst. I had treatments on Thursday mornings at 11:30. From the time I awoke, I was anxious. All morning, the anxiety would build. No one was home until my mom came by from work to pick me up. An hour or so before my mom arrived, I would get in the shower, turn the water on as hot as I could stand it, get into the fetal position, and cry. I would cry until I was choking for air. I would beg God to do anything to not let me have a treatment that day. There were times when I prayed that He would let me die so that I would not have to go to chemotherapy.

There were many times that I blamed God. How could He (or She or It) allow this to happen to me? What had I done to deserve this? I felt like I was in a hell far worse than I ever could have imagined.

I had been religious as a child and had attended Catholic school all of my life. After eighth grade, however, I started going to church less and less. By the time I finished high school, I was going to church on Christmas and sometimes Easter. I don't exactly know how I let this happen, but I did, and I didn't really miss going to church.

The first Sunday after I learned of my cancer diagnosis, I found myself back in church. I prayed and prayed. I asked for forgiveness and told God that I would do anything as long as He made this go away. I prayed for a miracle, but things just kept getting worse and worse. After a few weeks of going to church every Sunday, I stopped.

Do Bad Things Really Happen to Good People?

Up until I received my cancer diagnosis, I thought that everything made sense, that every question had an answer, and that there was a clear line between being a good person and a bad person. I believed that punishment was reserved for really bad people who deserved it. Or maybe, I just refused to accept that bad things happen to good people because it was something that I could not rationalize. I think these beliefs reflect how fortunate I had been in my life. No one close to me had died. Nothing really bad had ever happened to me or anyone else I loved. The major trauma in my life had been when my biology teacher gave me that B for the second semester of my freshman year of high school, and I realized that I would not be able to get straight A's. I had tried my best, and things hadn't worked out as I had wanted.

Being in and out of the hospital often, I had many roommates. I saw many people trapped in their own hells, and they were good people. Things stopped making sense. Lines started to blur. Questions stopped having answers.

I heard about my first roommate before I even met her. I had resumed baby-sitting a few days after I had finished all of the staging tests at the beginning of my cancer experience. I was determined to go back to work and pick up where I had left off. The people for whom I baby-sat needed to be convinced, but I told them I would be fine and that I could handle it. I somehow got through that day, but everything had changed. I was so tired. When I got home, I plopped down in front of the television.

On the television news was a report about a teenager who had been driving on the wrong side of the road and hit another car. The impact killed both people inside the other car. The teenager was in stable condition at the local hospital.

Just then the phone rang.

My mom answered it, and it was my doctor. All of my test results were in, and she wanted me to come back to the hospital that night so that the following morning I could undergo the last hurdle in the staging process—the surgery to biopsy my lymph nodes and organs. I was so mad. I was just starting to get my life back on track after the whole diagnosis. I resented my doctor for making one phone call and sending my life into complete chaos again.

I couldn't eat dinner. I felt this huge weight pressing in on me. Soon after, the doorbell rang. My friends wanted to know if I could come out for a while. Tearily, I explained that I had to go to the hospital. We talked for a while, and I remember thinking how lucky they were to be able to play until dark and go to bed in their own beds and wake up the next day at home. I hated that I was different. I hated that I had cancer.

I cried all the way to the hospital. I felt like once I entered that dreary building, it would somehow suck me up and I'd never get out alive. I had never before stayed in a hospital overnight. I walked into my room just as a doctor was pulling a long tube out of my roommate's lung. Her scream was the most horrible sound I had ever heard. It made me shiver, and for a moment I felt like bolting out the door and never coming back.

My roommate was being prepared for surgery. Soon after the tube was removed, the girl's parents and brother came back into the room. I hadn't even noticed them outside the door when I walked into the room. They gathered lovingly around her and said a family prayer.

A few days after my own surgery, I learned that the girl, my roommate for all of a half an hour, had been the one I had heard about on the news earlier that night—the one driving the car on the wrong side of the road who had killed two people. I had pictured "murderers" as horrible, selfish people who didn't care about those they had killed—not a scared teenager whose boyfriend stopped by to comfort her or whose family gathered around her and prayed. After her surgery, she was transferred to a different floor, but I later learned that she did not remember the accident, nor did she realize that she had killed two people.

When I got out of the intensive-care unit, I was put into a room with another roommate, a girl who had been in a terrible car accident. She was paralyzed on the right side of her body and couldn't talk. She was in diapers. All of her friends came to visit her. Day after day, I watched as her mom, dad, brother, grandmother, and school friends visited. To them, she was alive, and that's all that mattered.

Enter the next surgery, the next roommates. My roommates always gave me a sense of how life could, indeed, be worse. They left me asking, "What had these people done to deserve their fates? Did they (we) somehow deserve this suffering?"

After my first postcancer surgery, I was in a horrible mood. I felt like I had been double-whammied. I had gotten through the cancer, but now I was having trouble with my hips because of the massive dosages of steroids I had to take during treatment. When I came out of surgery, I wasn't medicated correctly, and it felt like someone was sawing through my left leg with a chain saw. A few hours later, the medication started to kick in, and I was transferred to my room. I was in a haze caused by the drugs and the pain.

As days passed and I became more alert, I happened to look out the door, and there stood an armed police officer. I thought, Oh, God, I must have been horrible when I came out of surgery. I vaguely recalled threatening to kill my doctor when he came in my room. I looked over at my roommate, who happened to sneeze at that moment. I noticed that she was handcuffed to the bed. My brother, always eager to get a rise out of me, called and asked, "How do you like your new roommate? I'd be careful at night if I were you." I later learned that she was serving time in a juvenile-detention center on weapons charges. She was having terrible pains in her leg, and the doctors discovered a benign tumor in her nerve. So then I thought, Okay, here is a criminal, and she gets off cancer-free. What in the heck did I ever do? I mean, if I was really horrible, wasn't the cancer punishment enough? One of the things that really struck me about my roommate, (besides the silver handcuff around her wrist) was that nobody ever came to visit her.

After another surgery, I didn't want to get up and walk around, nor would I touch my breathing device. These two techniques are supposed to keep a patient's lungs clear after surgery so that pneumonia doesn't set in. The boy in the room next to me had a similar surgery (although not cancer-related), and he was up and walking all of the time. The nurses kept telling me how well he was doing on his breathing exercises, trying to get a little friendly competition going, but I wasn't biting. I would have loved to have told them where they could have stuck those breathing devices. Two days later, he developed pneumonia, even though he did everything right. I also found out that his condition was terminal.

Even though I'm not sure about many aspects of religion, and I don't particularly feel "Catholic," I do believe in God. I know this may sound crazy, and I'm not sure how I'd react if I were a stranger reading this, but I have felt the presence of God in my life.

Halfway through my treatment, I gave up. I either refused to go to my chemo-therapy treatments, or I made it so difficult that my parents had to drag me there or police officers had to unlock doors that I had barricaded myself behind at the hospital. I wanted to live, but I couldn't take the treatments anymore, and without the treatments I would die. I stopped my treatments for two weeks in January, and I honestly believe that a presence larger than me or my parents, friends, or doctors brought me back—this is where I really felt that God was present for me, helping me to find the strength to resume treatments. I felt weak and as if I had let everyone down. I was really hard on myself, but as I have learned, there isn't a right way to fight cancer.

Why Do Some People Do Better Than Others?

Still, even after I beat cancer, the questions continued: Why am I here while others, who have fought harder than I have, aren't? Why are my hips screwed up while people who have had the exact same treatment as I did are fine? I don't think I'm stronger or fought harder than those who died. And I don't think that I have suffered more than people who haven't had cancer. I will admit, though, that there were times during my illness when I heard people complaining about things that I saw as petty and I wanted to say, "Get a grip!"

Everyone has his or her own sufferings; this is something that I learned during my experience. What amazes me is that, for the most part, you can never tell by just look-ing at a person what his or her suffering may be.

There was a time when I thought I had maxed out on suffering and that nothing could be as bad as having cancer. And then my grandmother died. It hurt like nothing I had ever felt before; it was a hurt different from cancer. And when my other grandmother passed away, I felt that hurt again. I wanted to believe that when one really bad thing happens in your life, that's it, you're done. I was so wrong.

Why Does Cancer Happen?

After years of struggling with these questions and months of trying to write this chapter, I decided to go to a family friend, who happens to be a priest, and discuss some of the issues that cancer brought, and still brings, into my life. I used to see priests as these mini-Gods—sort of how I thought that all of those Santas in the store at Christmas time somehow were related to the "real" Santa.

I met with the priest on the first day of spring. It was a cold, dreary day. It felt like spring was lost—sort of symbolic of how I'd been feeling spiritually. One of the many things I admire about this priest is that he is so easy to talk to. He never pretends to know something he doesn't, and he really listens to what people are saying. I asked him a series of questions about God, cancer, and suffering.

"As a recently diagnosed patient with cancer, I found that I often and truthfully struggle with the 'Why me?' question," I began. "At first, I thought of my illness as a punishment from God, even though I know that God doesn't and couldn't work this way. I guess what I am getting at is how would you respond to a teenager who is asking the 'Why me?' question or viewing his or her cancer as a punishment from God, or perhaps doing a bit of both?"

The priest replied, "From what I understand, these questions are good ones, and if I were in your spot I'd be asking the same questions. The key here is that these questions, although understandable, reveal a false idea of God. God does not punish. God is all-loving and has no desire to see people suffer. God is a healer—one who wants to hold all people in His arms. Over time, you can come to know God. Patience is the key. Terrible experiences can help you to learn who God is and see the role He plays in your life. If you wish to lash out, God understands. Always remember, God comes to those in need. Maybe it would be easier to think of God as a friend. Like any friendship, there are good times and bad times—times when everything is right and times when everything is wrong. A strong friendship requires patience, understanding, acceptance, struggle, and resolution. A strong relationship with God contains these elements, too."

Next, I asked the age-old question, "Why do bad things happen to good people?" I know there's a whole book on this question, but I really wanted to hear his take on it.

"I knew you were going to ask me this one," he said. "It's like we are trying to save God so He looks better. I struggle with this one, too. I cannot believe that God causes bad things because He is good and loving. I'd ask you to look at all the gifts in your life and then ask, 'Is this supposed to be a gift? Is there something I am supposed to learn from this?' I'm a creature of God. I'm dependent on God. My talents, my life are gifts from God. I am dependent on a Father who loves me very much. I'm good. God is good. This is bad. It's all about growing into who God is for you."

"It's hard for me to think I'm dependent on God and that my life isn't mine," I said. "Do you believe God gives people cancer?"

"No," the priest replied.

"But how can He allow cancer to happen?"

"Think about the worst trait of a person that you love," he said. "For example, say your mother is an alcoholic. You know your mother loves you. Does she drink because she doesn't love you?"

"Do you believe that everything happens for a reason?" I asked.

The priest replied, "I believe that everything can have a purpose. There is a process of getting through a difficult experience. At the end, you come to know things about yourself that you didn't know before. So often you can stand back once you have reached the other side and say, 'I know more about myself now.'"

I then asked what he would say to a teenager who was newly diagnosed with cancer. I used to hate it when people would say things to me like "God only gives you what you can handle" and "When God gives you a heavy load, He puts His hands under you to help carry you." Those remarks made me feel weak and guilty. If I was having a bad day and didn't feel much like fighting, I felt like I was failing—failing God.

He replied that he did not care for those types of remarks, either. He continued, "I would probably tell you I feel very badly for you. The road you are traveling is difficult, and I am not going to cheapen it or make less of the situation by saying, 'You'll be fine.' What I will do is pray for you. I'll be here for you. I'll do anything for you, just name it."

"Religion is a tough subject for me right now," I said. "I'm not sure where I stand on many issues. However, this is how I felt before I got cancer, and I haven't had a major change in my religious views after my cancer experience. I guess this surprises me. I figured I'd be either a religious fanatic or an atheist."

The priest replied, "Illnesses can make people very centered on themselves. You wake up in the morning and you think, 'Okay, how do I feel today? What do I have to do today to fight my illness?' But think about when you are happiest. It's when you can get away from yourself. Maybe you are out with friends at a concert or on vacation. It's hard to measure up when you are in a constant battle with yourself. I'm trying to say that an illness can make you so focused on yourself and zap you of any leftover energy. During a period of illness, it can be hard to change other aspects of your life such as spiritual beliefs. You're doing all you can just to hang on."

What Can I Learn From It All?

My conversation with the priest started me thinking: Could I somehow locate a priest who had cancer as a teenager? This priest was always very careful to point out that he never had cancer and, therefore, could not fully understand what I was going through. As it turned out, I didn't have to look very far at all. I happened to be reading an old issue of my college's quarterly magazine when I saw, right there on the front page, a story about a priest at my college who had been treated for leukemia as a young adult. I made a few phone calls and within two weeks was on campus having a conversation with him.

I wasn't really sure how to conduct the interview because I had so many questions, so I asked him to tell me about his cancer experience. It was as if he knew every question that I was going to ask him because he ended up answering all of my questions before I had even asked a single one.

In 1973, he was diagnosed with leukemia. He was in eighth grade. He remembers starting to play a game of football in his yard and quickly discovering that he could not run the length of the yard without becoming exhausted. He went inside and told his parents that he was too tired to play football. His parents told him to go to bed. The next morning, while fixing breakfast, he was overcome by the heat from the oven and collapsed. His parents took him to the emergency room.

He soon found himself undergoing several tests, after which the diagnosis was clear: leukemia. For four years, he underwent chemotherapy and radiation. He describes the treatment as "horrific." During his sophomore year of high school, he lost his hair because of the radiation treatments. He bought a wig at a store named Wigs-N-Things. With a half-smirk on his face, Father recalled a time in school when he got in trouble for talking. As the teacher came toward him, he twisted his wig on his head, which made the teacher back off.

This priest is a first-generation childhood cancer survivor. He told me that he once looked up *leukemia* in the *World Book Encyclopedia* only to discover the words "fatal disease" under it.

He has learned much from his cancer experience. He sees every day as a gift. He has a deeper appreciation of life and a heightened awareness of God's presence in life. He also has experienced the depth of his parents' love, a love he shares with nine other siblings. I could totally relate to what he was saying about having the experience of fully understanding how much parents love their children.

At different times throughout my treatment, both of my parents told me that they wished it were them instead of me. They'd switch places with me in a minute if they could. That awed me because they saw how much pain I was in and how sick I got, and they would rather suffer themselves than to have me suffer. That is unconditional love. As I told the priest this, he nodded and said his parents had said the same things to him.

Father said that his parents always wanted him to remember that there were good things in the world even though what he was going through was bad. His parents always countered something bad with something good. He remembers going out for an ice cream cone after undergoing a bone marrow test. He also got to sit in the pilot's seat of a Cessna aircraft.

His parents didn't want him to know that he had cancer. They told him that he was anemic. However, his doctor felt that he should know and told him one day, as he was receiving radiation.

As a child, he wasn't particularly religious. When he was diagnosed with cancer, he never felt that God was punishing or testing him. He always knew he would survive. He laughed when he said, "My mother always looked at the worst possible thing that could happen in any given situation. That way, she was ready for the worst even though the worst seldom happened. My mother had my grave picked out."

I told him that I hated when people said things to me like, "God only gives you what you can handle." He nodded and said, "What God gives us is the grace to handle what life gives us."

He said he wants teens who are undergoing cancer treatment to know that God is ever-present with them and that this is not something that God did to them. He says to ask God for the gifts of strength and hope; God, cure me, but in the meantime give me strength.

He concluded by saying, "I don't think there is a reason why people get cancer. It's just how life works. God created the world, and in this world there is disease and tragedy. One person in a million wins the lottery. People get terrible illnesses. God is present within all of this."

The part of our conversation that really struck me was when Father talked about faith. "Faith has a huge role in how a person deals with suffering," he said. "Faith gives hope and meaning to one's suffering. The core of suffering is being alone, but with faith we come to understand that we are not alone."

What I Know For Sure

- I do believe in God (which I think I always knew but maybe somehow just forgot).
- I learned much by talking with two people of great faith.
- Cancer has brought many good things into my life, although until a few years ago, I would have never believed it.
- I had a genuine appreciation for each day when I was sick—something I had never known before my cancer, nor have been able to quite recapture since my remission.
- I am so happy to be alive (even on the bad days).

Chapter 7.

You Mean I Still Have to Go to School?

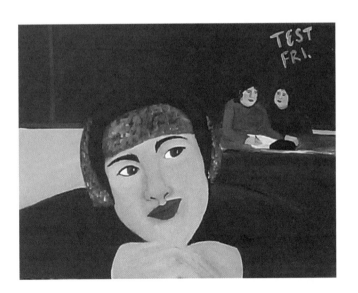

Chapter 7.

You Mean I Still Have to Go to School?

When I started my sophomore year of high school, I was halfway through my first chemotherapy cycle. Three or four of the people I went to school with knew that I had cancer because I had been in touch with them over the summer. My principal and all of the teachers also knew because my parents called and talked to the principal who, in turn, talked with the teachers.

Personally, I was relieved that my principal and teachers knew. From the beginning, they were supportive, and I felt that we were able to openly communicate about problems and concerns as they arose.

I didn't really know how to tell my classmates. I missed the entire second week of school, and people naturally started asking me questions. I told them that I had a bad case of the flu. But then, I really started to lose my hair and was missing more and more school.

With my permission, the school psychologist talked to my classmates about my cancer. I was out sick that day, but I felt that it was important to gather everyone together and tell them all the facts. This way, rumors were prevented before they could start.

I feel that school was one of the things that kept me going during those long months of chemotherapy. My classmates were wonderful, always asking how I was and eager to help me with assignments. My teachers also helped me in every way they could. At school, I felt normal—or at least as close to normal as possible. After all, that's where a 16-year-old is supposed to be during the day. Sitting in a classroom beats sitting in a hospital waiting room anticipating chemotherapy.

I had to take a leave from school during the last two months of my sophomore year. At this time, I met with teachers individually to complete the remainder of my assignments.

Again, I would never want to sound like my opinion or experience is the only approach to a situation. While doing research for the book, I came across a booklet titled *Help Yourself: Tips for Teenagers With Cancer,* which is a free publication offered by the National Cancer Institute, 1980. Following are a couple of excerpts that deal with school.

"Although I didn't want to talk about my cancer in front of the whole class, I did want to tell a few people. I felt a lot better after I talked to them."—Barbara (p. 30)

"I asked other teenagers with cancer what they were doing about going back to school. Then considered my own position on it and decided for myself. At school I have more friends to talk to and I am happier. I went back as soon as I could." —Ron (p. 31)

You may be missing some school because of your treatment. Or, you may not feel like going to school for many reasons. However, it is important to keep going to school if at all possible. Learning is your "job" right now. Even though you have cancer, you still need to prepare yourself for work or college, just like anyone else. It is also important to be around people your own age. In my opinion, preparing for the future helps someone believe in his or her future. It also gives a person a sense of control that otherwise may be overshadowed by cancer.

School Tips

If you know you'll be out of school for a long time, you and your parents may be able to arrange for a home tutor. You also can work out an arrangement with your regular teachers or with students in your classes to bring your assignments home to you.

When it's time to go back into the classroom, talk to your counselor, school nurse, or teacher. Include your parents and someone from the treatment center in your meeting if it would make you feel more comfortable. Together, you can plan your schedule and assignments and discuss what to tell your classmates.

Because your school peers may have questions about your illness, you may want to have someone from the school or treatment center talk to your class: "A man named Mr. Reeder was a guidance counselor at my school. His mother had cancer, and he knew what I had, so he told the student body. I didn't mind."—Ron (NCI, 1980, p. 31)

Others would rather not do this. Barbara, who is quoted at the beginning of the chapter, preferred to simply tell a few friends about her cancer and then answer questions as they came up.

When you miss school, keeping up with the work can be difficult. Try to work out a schedule and assignments with your teachers so that you aren't constantly behind. If you set your study goals and meet them—in spite of treatment—you'll feel good about yourself and your schoolwork.

Some Problems That I Faced at School and How I Solved Them

Problem One

I used to go to school for a half-day before my chemotherapy treatment. I hated missing school and wanted to be there as much as possible. At 11:30 am, I went to the school office, where my mom picked me up for treatment. As this time drew nearer, I became more anxious. One day I was trying to take a French quiz at 11 am. I was so anxious about going to the hospital that I went totally blank and couldn't finish the quiz. I knew the quiz was on easy material, and that made me even more upset. After my French class was over, I went to my teacher and explained what happened. She said she'd let me make it up at another time. Most teachers are understanding and willing to help you in any way they can. You just need to talk to them about what you are going through. The scenario I just described made me realize that it would be better to stay at home on the morning of my chemotherapy treatments because I was so anxious that I could not concentrate in school.

Problem Two

My school had a dress code, and before I got my wig, I needed to do something to cover my head because my hair was really thinning. One day, I wore a scarf around my head, and one of my classmates began to harass me about defying the dress code. I was saddened and upset by her remarks until I realized that she did not know that I had cancer.

It is hard to decide what to do when a situation like this occurs. I just walked away from her. A few weeks later, when the psychologist talked to my class, the classmate came back and apologized to me. She just didn't know.

Problem Three

I often felt isolated and alone at school. I wished I had the problems that my peers were experiencing. I felt left out because I frequently was sick on Friday nights because of my Thursday chemotherapy treatments and couldn't attend the football games and other social events.

I needed to realize that the problems my classmates were experiencing were very real problems for them. They would have been my problems, too, if cancer hadn't entered the picture and complicated my life. I joined in activities and outings when I felt well enough. I had to realize that there would be more football games and social activities.

Problem Four

My doctor suggested that I not participate in gym class. I talked with my gym teacher. I went to gym class with my class and watched or did things that required minimal physical activity or contact, like keeping score. We found supplemental projects for me to do in order to get credit for the class.

Problem Five

I often felt behind and overwhelmed with the amount of work I missed. I felt like I was going to have to repeat my sophomore year of high school.

I talked with my teachers and made schedules as to when my assignments needed to be completed. I also took my assignments one by one when I felt well enough to do them. I realized that while school is important, getting better is more important.

I also tried to set short-term goals for myself. It gave me something to aim for, and I felt like I accomplished something when I achieved my goal. However, I had to make my goals realistic or I would be setting myself up for failure. I also tried to remember to mix school work and fun when I felt well enough.

As it turned out, each student in my English class was required to keep a journal during the year I was sick. I want to share some of my entries because I think they authentically capture how I was feeling at certain times. Journaling may help you to deal with your situation.

Wednesday, September 6, 1989

I am so sick of being sick. All I do is sit around all day and throw up. I am so bored that I want to scream. I hate missing school, and I know that when I do eventually get back that I'll have major work to do. Of course, there was no way that I could go in today unless they wanted to wheel me around on a stretcher with a puke dish in my hand. I know that must sound pretty gross, but that is the way I feel. I can't even believe that I am saying this, but I am sick of television—all of those perky, beautiful, healthy actors and actresses.

Wednesday, September 20, 1989

I am so glad that I don't have to go to the hospital this Thursday. Finally, my first really free weekend since school started. I have no idea what I want to do, but it has to be something exciting.

Tuesday, September 26, 1989

I'm pretty happy today. I got a 40/42 on my geometry test. Even though I'm happy, the thought of going in for chemotherapy on Thursday is still in the back of my mind. It is always there. I keep trying to remind myself that life will go on after Thursday, and I will have one more treatment under my belt.

Sunday, October 1, 1989

All I have done today is homework, and I really haven't gotten very far. On Thursday, I am going in for chemotherapy, and on Tuesday the 10th, I'm going to have my Mediport put in. In other words, surgery. My hair is so thin, and I wonder if my life is ever going to get better. I feel like I am going to die. I wish I could be like my friends. They baby-sit on the weekends, love school, and have their health.

Wednesday, October 25, 1989

I am sitting in English class right now writing this journal. I am starting to feel a little less sick. I am always so relieved when I start feeling better because when I am really sick, it feels like it is never going to end. My friend and I were just discussing our French skit. I am responsible for turning the tape on at the right time. My friend said something like, "We gave you an easy part because we didn't know if you'd be here." Even though I understand, my feelings were still hurt. I don't want people to lower their standards for me.

Tuesday, November 2, 1989

I am so tired, and I have a huge World History test tomorrow. I am sort of excited because I have a baby-sitting job on Saturday. I really miss being able to baby-sit regularly like I used to. I'm so glad they called me, and I'm so glad that I don't have chemo this week.

Tuesday, November 21, 1989

I got a pleasant surprise today. Chemo was postponed because my blood counts were low, and Thanksgiving is saved. I can't go back to school until I get my blood retested a week from Thursday. I'm sort of happy for the break. I'm going to sleep and get caught up on my homework.

Wednesday, December 13, 1989

I am starting to get excited about Christmas. My cousin is coming in from California. I am asking for a waterbed, but I don't know if I'll get it. My older brother is coming home from college tomorrow. I'm looking forward to seeing him.

Monday, December 25, 1989

Christmas. Even though today was a great day, I kept thinking, I hope this isn't my last Christmas.

Wednesday, January 3, 1990

I was just thinking about all of the things that have happened during the past year. On the good side, I became a godmother, and I got my kitten, Darby. On the bad side, well, cancer and my aunt died.

Saturday, January 27, 1990

Today was a great day. I went out to lunch with my dad, grandmother, and older brother. I went to my friend's birthday party and met her two cute cousins. I went home and a couple of my friends from school called. I had pizza for dinner. My friend called and asked me to come over and visit her while she was baby-sitting. I walked all the way around the block and wasn't even tired. I had a nice visit with my friend and the kids. Today, I just felt so lucky to not be sick. Yes, I will be sick next Saturday, but I am not sick today.

Tuesday, February 13, 1990

I am really fed up. I am behind in school, treatments, and life in general. As hard as I try to get my life back to normal, it seems that I am failing badly. I can't accept this disease. I'd do anything to delay my treatments even though I know I need them to get better and by delaying them I am only prolonging them. Sometimes I'll just be sitting there and it's like, "God, I have cancer." I wish I had hair to brush. No one seems to understand.

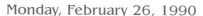

Monday, February 26, 1990

Well, at least my mom and dad are happy. Katie was a good girl and didn't fight the doctors. I am so sick of everything and totally pissed off.

Monday, March 26, 1990

Sophomore dance was okay. My date didn't really want to dance. Actually, that was fine with me because I've been so tired lately. We sat at a table and talked with other couples. That was fun. I wonder if I'll ever get married and have children?

Tuesday, April 3, 1990

I haven't been sleeping very well because of a medicine that I am taking. I've been watching a lot of late-night television. I also have an incredible appetite and have been eating everything in sight. I get these really insane cravings. Last night it was ribs. Today in school I would have killed for cheese popcorn.

Tuesday, May 15, 1990

After talking with my school counselor, we decided that it would be best if I completed the rest of the school year at home. I have just been so sick. The other day I was having problems just sitting up in class. She told me, "You're going to make it through your sophomore year, kiddo." I smiled. Trust me, there were times when I didn't think I would. I just have a few more assignments and projects to complete, and then I will be a junior.

Victory

In June of 1992, after a year and a half of remission, one hip surgery down, and one to go, I graduated from high school with my class.

It's weird to describe what high school was to me. My freshman and senior years were what I'd call normal. The two years in between, though—wow! There were great times—dances, football games, memorable times with friends, and there were awful times, too, and there was always cancer.

National Cancer Institute. (1980). *Help yourself: Tips for teenagers with cancer.* Bethesda: Author.

Chapter 8.

What Other Young Adult Cancer Survivors Have to Say

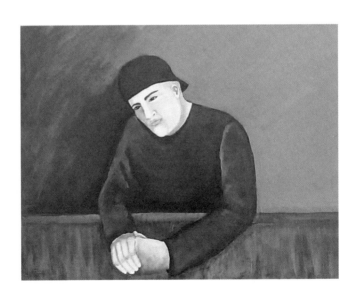

Chapter 8.

What Other Young Adult Cancer Survivors Have to Say

To me, this is the most important chapter of the book. It's what I consider to be the heart of the book.

As I began to write this book, I realized that I didn't want it to just be the story of one 16-year-old with Hodgkin's disease. I wanted it to be about other young people who have experienced cancer, gotten through it, and gone on with their lives. So, I set out on a personal mission—to find people who had experienced cancer as a teenager. I developed a Web page on the Internet, contacted people listed in pen pal lists through the Candlelighters Childhood Cancer Foundation, and asked doctors send out letters to former patients about my project.

Soon, people began responding. People who didn't even know me somehow trusted me enough to openly share their cancer experiences so that they could help others. I thank each of them because there wouldn't be a book without them.

This chapter consists of the personal stories of 24 people who had cancer when they were young. Each story is unique and special. I often have said that when I was diagnosed with cancer, I felt like I was the only teenager in the universe going through it. I hope this chapter will help you to see that you are not alone.

Twenty-Four Cancer Journeys

Jane Beckett

Type of cancer: Ovarian cancer
Age at diagnosis: 7
Current age: 29
Occupation: Massage therapist
Jane's advice: The main thing is to ask questions about your disease, the treatment, and any side effects. There is no such thing as a silly or embarrassing question when it concerns you or your body. Laugh and cry a lot.

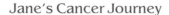

Jane's Cancer Journey

My first remembrance that something was wrong was at the end of a school day. It seemed like suddenly, my stomach began to feel like it was twisting around. I really wanted to see the nurse, but my second-grade teacher wouldn't let me because we were about to be dismissed for the day. I had to wait until I got home. It was only about an eight-block walk home, but at the time, it seemed to go on forever. I cried all the way home, holding my belly because it hurt so much. When I finally reached my doorstep, I can remember flinging my books on the floor and dropping and rolling around on the floor, crying.

The next thing I knew, I was being whisked to my pediatrician's office and then to the hospital. There, I didn't feel any pain, so I figured everything was okay. I don't remember the tests they did at this hospital, but apparently they did plenty of them and could find nothing. I still was having pain when they palpated my lower abdomen.

Because the tests came up inconclusive, the next step was exploratory surgery. I was seven years old and had no clue as to what was going on—I was just happy to be out of school. The surgeon happened to be a family friend from church. I think this made my parents feel a little more at ease.

I remember waiting to go to surgery and coloring a picture. A nurse came by and said that I should be very proud because I was the only one who stayed inside the lines. Next thing I knew, they were wheeling me into the operating room, and that's when I lost it—hysterical crying, screaming, kicking, the works. My doctor said that if I didn't calm down, he'd give me something to really cry about. I hyperventilated so much that I think I sucked in a little too much anesthesia. Right now, as I'm thinking about it, I can still taste the anesthesia.

What they found was a shock to everyone.

A tumor had wrapped itself around my left ovary and killed it. The pain I had been feeling was the ovary being twisted by the tumor. The hardest part, I remember after the surgery, was sitting up. As soon as I did, it felt like the stitches were ripping out of me. I wish someone had told me about the importance of keeping up your abdominal strength then. Once I was cleared to go home, all thoughts went to a Burger King® cheeseburger. Hospital food was not my favorite.

I thought everything had been taken care of and that I was free of doctors' poking. My mom said that I asked why they didn't go ahead and take the other ovary while they where in there. I wasn't going to have kids, anyway! Apparently, I began to show similar symptoms a few months later. I experienced extreme fatigue, to the point of opting for a nap rather than playing with my friends; irritability; and minor cuts and bruises that took a long time to heal. That's when Memorial Sloan-Kettering Cancer Center came into the picture. My main concerns were missing school and going to New York City. Little did I know that I was going to become a specimen. It seemed like I just went from one doctor to the next. Everybody wanted a blood sample. I was always waiting to see what kind of test I had to go through. To this day, when someone mentions giving blood, my arms automatically go up in defense. Endless blood tests, computerized tomography (CT) scans, gallium scans, enemas, and the smell of my doctor's cologne—these are my first memories of New York.

I guess I realized that something pretty serious was going on when I noticed that I was the only kid around with hair. No matter where I went in the hospital, it seemed like I was the only one without a scarf or a cap covering a bald head.

Again, it was decided that surgery was the next step. The tests didn't really show anything positive or negative, but the doctors needed to look inside and make sure nothing had spread. After that surgery, I remember seeing my mom and dad standing by the window and crying. I thought to myself, Why are they crying? I'm right here. I'm okay. I can't imagine what was going through their minds. All I knew was that in my mind, I had made it through the surgery, and if I had done that, then things were good. Luckily, thanks to a tremendous amount of prayer and family support, that was the case.

I had to go back every three months, then six months, and then once a year for five years for checkups. After receiving that final clean bill of health, I think my entire family gave a collective sigh of relief.

I don't know who was looking over me during that time, but I am very grateful that they were. There were times when I felt scared and not sure of what was going on, but I really feel blessed that I had no idea how severe things were or might have become. I wasn't spending too much time worrying about things that I really didn't understand.

That feeling has carried over into my profession. I'm a massage therapist in a chiropractic clinic. I see individuals who worry so much about things that are beyond their control that it puts my own fears about things into perspective. I know what I can and cannot control, and I have to be willing to deal with whatever comes my way.

It sounds very easy, but I have wonderful support from my family and friends. They have no problem setting me straight when a problem arises.

Troy Braden

Type of cancer: Germinoma brain tumor
Age at diagnosis: 17
Current age: 20
Occupation: Student
Troy's advice: Don't keep your emotions bottled up. Share how you are feeling with friends and family because it will help you feel better.

Troy's Cancer Journey

I was diagnosed with a brain tumor in May 1996. My family and I were shocked. Just one year prior to my cancer diagnosis, I was told that I had a digestive disorder called Crohn's disease.

My brain tumor was a little bigger than a golf ball, and it had cut off circulation in the ventricles of my brain by pinching them shut. As a result, I developed hydrocephalus. This means that I had an abnormal amount of fluid in my skull.

My doctors were unable to remove the tumor surgically, so they took a biopsy and drained the excess fluid from my ventricles. I then had chemotherapy treatments to shrink the tumor. As a result of the treatment, I became very worn down and slept often. I had blood transfusions to help to alleviate my fatigue. I didn't have much of an appetite and lost weight, going from 138 to 99 pounds. The good news was that my tumor was shrinking. After I finished all of my chemotherapy sessions, I began radiation therapy. This was harder on me than the chemotherapy had been. I was sick all of the time. Whenever I think of radiation, I think of nuclear bombs and, obviously, death.

Eventually, the tumor was gone. Now, I return to the hospital about every two months for blood work and an occasional magnetic resonance imaging scan.

I still worry about the tumor coming back, but I know I have to move on. I start college in a couple of months and hope someday to become a child life specialist. I want to give back a little of the love and hope that I received.

Marshall Buckley

Type of cancer: Hodgkin's disease
Age at diagnosis: 14
Current age: 16
Occupation: Student
Marshall's advice: Do everything in your power to keep your mind off the chemo while you get it—that includes not looking at it (especially doxorubicin, the red stuff!).

Marshall's Cancer Journey

Cancer. The forbidden word. At least that's what most people tend to make of it. But yet, it's all around us. Nearly every day, you hear about it in one way or another. And naturally, everyone takes his or her good health for granted, until a loved one develops cancer, or, the most horrifying of all—*you develop it.*

I can remember when I was a kid, my brother used to play with all of his toy cars. Every so often, he would play with his toy ambulance, pretending there was some type of emergency. He would say something like, "Oh no! He has cancer." I never thought much of that until recently.

It all started when I finished taking a shower one night. For some reason, I noticed two lumps in my neck. It freaked me out because I could see them popping out of my skin. I didn't know what the heck was going on, and neither did my mom. We waited until the next day to go to my doctor. I had just gotten over a bad case of bronchitis a week or two before. Since that time, I had been having trouble with my breathing, and sometimes I felt light-headed. I also had experienced two separate occasions of night sweats.

When I went to see the doctor, he told me the bumps were my lymph nodes, but he was puzzled as to why they were like that. He ordered blood work and a chest x-ray, but even those results weren't clear. I had a whole mass in the area of my lungs and heart, and the doctor thought that I had a bad case of pneumonia or even tuberculosis. He sent me to get a CT scan the next day.

That's when all the bad things began to happen.

I soon found myself being transferred to a nationally known hospital. There, my new doctor thoroughly explained everything that was happening. I was scared and sick to my stomach, but still I had an interest in the things they were doing to me.

It wasn't until after everything was done that I came to hate all they did to me.

When I was in the hospital, I noticed everything that was going on. They put me in the intensive-care unit the first night because I was having trouble breathing. I found intensive care pretty interesting because they had to hook up all these patches to me and connect them to a big monitor. I held my breath intentionally, and the computer would sound this alarm, which would call the nurse. That night, I was also surprised to find that my choir director had come to see how I was doing. This showed me that he really cared about his students, and it helped me a great deal through that first week in the hospital.

After my night in intensive care, I underwent surgery to stage my cancer. My full diagnosis: Hodgkin's disease stage IVB NS. The IVB part meant that I was in stage four (there are four stages of Hodgkin's disease) and that I had symptoms of the disease (B means symptomatic, A means no symptoms). The NS (nodular sclerosing) is the cell type. Later, I found out that if I hadn't gone into the hospital, I probably would have been dead in three days. That really hit me hard.

My treatments consisted of six cycles of chemotherapy. There were two sessions in each cycle. I can remember back to the day in the hospital when I got my first treatment. Soon after I began to get it, I started to feel queasy.

The beginning of the treatments was like having the flu. I was sick to my stomach, and different foods began to make me sick even when I thought of them. Another thing that really bothered me was the drug, doxorubicin. It is red. All I did was look at it, and I felt like I was going to vomit. One of its side effects is that it turns the urine red.

As time went on, I discovered that if I could keep my mind off the chemotherapy, I could make myself feel a little better. I also found something to set my mind on. I heard about the Make-A-Wish Foundation, an organization that grants wishes to kids with life-threatening diseases. The only thing I wanted was a computer. I had always wanted a computer.

And sure enough, my wish was granted.

I'll never forget the day I came home, and there were three cars in my driveway. I walked into my bedroom, and all I could see were big boxes. I had gotten my very own computer, and I couldn't have been happier.

After I was done with chemotherapy, I still had to go through radiation therapy. There was about a two-month lapse between the time I finished chemo and when I started radiation. During that period, I came down with shingles and had to be hospitalized for three days so that I could receive medicines intravenously.

After the shingles were cured, I had to undergo radiation therapy five days a week for a month straight. When my radiation treatments were over, I was considered to be in remission. But it wasn't over.

I ended up going through post-traumatic stress syndrome. This is the time when everything hit me, and it hit really hard. I went through a great deal of commotion with my parents and with many other things around me. I fell into a deep depression, and it kept getting worse. One of the side effects I experienced was panic attacks. It was as if I became a totally different person caused by all the built-up anger and stress inside of me. A lot of that anger had to do with cancer and why I had to go through it. It got so bad that, at one point, I felt like I didn't want to live anymore.

It was like the world was going through a nuclear war and everyone was destroyed but me. I was left to suffer, and there was no one to help. I didn't feel like living because it seemed like there was no hope. I felt that way for quite a while. It was like I got kicked out the back door after treatment and was left to start over all by myself.

Fortunately, I got professional help, and today I'm on my way back up.

Dianne Chapman

Type of cancer: Dysgerminoma (ovarian cancer)
Age at diagnosis: 16
Current age: 26
Occupation: Teacher at a daycare
Dianne's advice: Believe in yourself and trust that God will pull you through.

Dianne's Cancer Journey

I had dysgerminoma or, in nonmedical terms, ovarian cancer. I had an easier time with my treatment because I was 16 and wanted children later in life. My doctors tried to do as little as possible. I chose to have surgery and then have my doctors watch me closely.

I had three different doctors in a week and a half, blood tests every day, and a bunch of other tests. In surgery, they removed my ovary and fallopian tube on the left side. I was so scared to go into surgery. I was eight when I had my first operation; I tore my liver in a car accident. This time, I was all alone and far from home. I was living in California at the time and visiting my aunt in Washington. I spent a week in the hospital all alone. My parents came to visit, but they could only stay a few hours, and they took my sister back with them.

My cancer was completely contained in my ovary, so my doctors were really hopeful that they got it all and it wouldn't come back. If it did, they were going to use more aggressive treatment. I would then have to have another surgery and have chemotherapy and radiation.

We all trusted the doctor, but he wanted us to get a second opinion just to give us other options. He sent us to a medical center in California, where the doctor wanted to treat me like a lab experiment. He wanted to give me chemo and radiation, then one year after my surgery do another operation just so he could look around inside of me. He didn't even care how I felt about it. It didn't even matter to him if I wanted children or not. He was going to do what he wanted and what he felt was right.

Two years after my cancer surgery, my doctors discovered another tumor. Everyone was afraid that my cancer had come back. I went through the same tests I had before, but it wasn't cancer. It's been 10 years since my diagnosis, and I have had no major problems. I am now 26 years old.

Bethany Columbus

Type of cancer: Acute lymphoblastic leukemia (ALL with a chromosome change)
Age at diagnosis: 12
Current age: 14
Occupation: Student
Bethany's advice: Believe in yourself, and you will make it.

Bethany's Cancer Journey

It all started when the health nurses came to vaccinate the kids at my school with the hepatitis B vaccine. After I had the vaccination, I always seemed to have sinus colds. I didn't go to the doctor because I thought, Well, it's winter, and lots of people have colds.

March break came, and I went to my aunt's house with my brother to stay for a couple of nights. When I came home, I was really stuffed up, and every time I blew my nose, there was blood. I thought it was because my aunt's house is really dry and she smokes. Then one day, my mom took me to the doctor because my skin looked yellow. My doctor said I had blood in my nose because I was constantly blowing it and that I was yellow from blowing so much. The doctor also said I had a sinus cold and put me on antibiotics. They seemed to help, but once I was off of the antibiotics, the sinus cold came back.

In April, I was due for another hepatitis B shot. I was still sick, and I remembered that my health teacher said if you were sick that you shouldn't get your vaccine. I told my mom about what my health teacher said. My mom wrote a note saying that I was sick and that it was up to my health teacher's discretion. My teacher said I would be fine and threw the note out. So that day, I received the vaccine.

That Friday, as I was coming out of the car after I finished power skating, I hit the side of my leg on the door. That night, I looked at my leg and saw a very big bruise. Saturday came, and I went power skating again. I was having a hard time keeping up because I was very tired. Then I felt really sick and threw up. I went home early, and on the way home my dad said he was embarrassed and that I would never make it at anything because I was a quitter. That same day we bought some trees and planted them in the rain. I was so weak and tired, but no one would believe me. They thought I was just being lazy.

On Sunday, I went outside to play with my brother and our friends. While they built a fort, I could only sit and watch. I started to get thirsty, so I went with one of my friends to my house to get a drink. When we were walking, I felt my stomach, and it seemed bigger than normal and hard. I passed my mom and dad on the way. I showed my mom my stomach, but she didn't say anything.

My friend and I got to my house and had a drink, but then my friend had to go home. I was home by myself when my stomach started to hurt really bad. I lay on the floor and hoped it would go away, but it didn't. My cat, Nelson, was meowing and wouldn't leave my side. I was crying. I thought about going to find my parents and telling them that I needed to go to the hospital, but I thought my dad would get upset if it ended up being nothing. Times before, I went to the hospital with stomach aches and they were nothing. Then the pains got worse, and I decided I needed to find my parents.

Crying, I went outside. My neighbor asked me what was wrong, and I told him. Together, we went to find my parents. My dad asked me what was wrong. I told him that my stomach really hurt and that I needed to go to the hospital. He said they would probably take some of my blood. I knew they would.

When I got to the hospital, they took some blood and did some x-rays. They found out that both of my knees were fractured; this was caused by the cells in my marrow cramming together. I had to stay in the hospital overnight. The doctor thought it could be mono or hepatitis, but he decided to send me to a specialist at a different hospital. I was only at that hospital for four hours before I was moved to a different hospital where I was diagnosed with acute lymphoblastic leukemia.

I had a feeling I had leukemia because I heard some nurses talking about it in the hall. I told my dad that I thought I had leukemia and that I might even die. Then the doctor came in and told me I had leukemia. He asked me if I knew what it was and what can happen. All I knew is that I would lose my hair.

My treatments started, and I had some really hard times. I had to have surgery to have fluid drained from my right side, where an infection developed. When I woke up, I had a chest tube and one of my ribs had been removed. The infection got into the lining of my lung and one of my ribs. After surgery, I was really hungry. Not knowing I had lost a rib, I asked someone to go to a restaurant and get me some ribs. Everyone thought that was funny.

On my birthday, I got bad news from my doctor. The doctor told my parents I needed a bone marrow transplant. My mom, dad, and brother all were tested to see if they were a match, but none of them were. People we knew and people from different churches all over the world got tested. We wanted to find a donor as quick as possible because I had a chromosome change, which could make me relapse.

Luckily, a donor was found for me in seven weeks. All I know about my donor is that he is male and a six out of six match for me. I had a high-dose chemotherapy treatment and three days of full-body radiation, twice a day, which was done to destroy my bone marrow. It wasn't long before I was in an isolation room. I couldn't step on the floor unless there was a towel there. There was no bathroom; I had to go in a commode chair.

Soon, I had my transplant, and there was nothing to it. In fact, I slept through most of it. It was just like getting blood. After it, we were all waiting for my white blood cell counts to come up. The doctors said that a person remains in the transplant unit from 14 to 25 days, at which point the counts are high enough so the person can go to a step-down hospital unit and then home. At day 27, I was still in the transplant unit, and my doctors started to worry that the bone marrow transplant wasn't working. They thought they might have to do another transplant. My family and I were upset by this. I prayed that my counts would go up, and so did many other people. I guess it worked because that very day, my counts starting coming up and they stayed up. On day 33, I got to go to a step-down unit. After being in bed for so long, I had to learn to walk again. I also had some problems with high blood pressure and high blood sugar levels, but these problems are now gone.

I can walk. I have lots of hair. I am feeling wonderful.

Amity Jolaine Cordell

Type of cancer: Thyroid cancer
Age at diagnosis: 12
Current age: 16
Occupation: High school student
Amity's advice: Believe in God and He will carry you through whatever you are facing. You have to believe that you can make it, and you will.

Amity's Cancer Journey

When I was 12 years old, I was diagnosed with thyroid cancer. On Wednesday, February 8, 1995, my doctor did a biopsy, taking a sample of a lump in the middle of my neck. That Friday, the doctor called my mom at work and told her that I had cancer. On March 15, 1995, I went into the hospital for surgery. The doctor thought that it would only take a few hours, but it ended up taking five-and-one-half hours, and I spent eight days in the hospital.

I have a scar that goes from one ear right across to the other ear. The left side of my neck and my left ear are still numb because the doctor had to cut nerves when he made the incision.

After the surgery, I had to go back into the hospital for an internal form of radiation known as radioactive iodine therapy. I spent three days and two nights in a room by myself. Because of the internal form of radiation that was used, my parents were only allowed to take two or three steps into my room to avoid being exposed to the radiation. They were not allowed to touch or hug me. That was the hardest and saddest part of all.

Barbara Cuccovia

Type of cancer: Hodgkin's disease
Age at diagnosis: 16
Current age: 23
Occupation: Nurse
Barbara's advice: Take your days one at a time. Be involved in your care by asking questions and making decisions. Most of all, remember to be a teenager and live your life.

Barbara's Cancer Journey

I was diagnosed with Hodgkin's disease when I was 16. I had found a lump on my chest and ignored it for about a week, thinking it was just that, a lump. When the bump didn't go away, I showed it to my mom. We then went to see my pediatrician about it.

I got an x-ray, which showed a mass. At that moment, I knew it was a tumor. I was extremely frightened and nervous because my pediatrician was talking to my mom and not to me. The pediatrician sent us to an oncologist who was honest from the beginning and did not sugarcoat what was happening. He immediately sent me for blood work and a CT scan. I was admitted to the hospital two days later for a biopsy, which confirmed a diagnosis of Hodgkin's disease.

I decided, at that point, that I was going to beat this thing and that it was not going to stop me from being me. I endured eight months of chemotherapy and, throughout this time, went to school, held a part-time job, and played lacrosse. Since June 30, 1992, I have been "cured."

This disease became a part of my life and has played a major role in who I am today. I am 23 years old and a nurse at New York University Medical Center. I became a nurse because I found the nurse who worked with my oncologist to be the most amazing person. I hope to be a nurse like her. I work on an adult medical floor, but after I have one year of experience, I plan to move into pediatrics. My goal is to become a pediatric oncology nurse and give back all that was given to me.

Marc Dewey

Type of cancer: Chronic myeloid leukemia
Age at diagnosis: 19
Current age: 30
Occupation: Radiation therapist
Marc's advice: Keep your head and heart up. Be an active participant in your care. Take control when it fits and accept help and support at other times. Appreciate the sunshine in your everyday life. Take care and live well.

Marc's Cancer Journey

Leukemia is a serious and life-threatening illness that, in varying forms, can affect a person at any age. Chronic myeloid leukemia, CML, is a particular strand of leukemia that will have great bearing on this story, as it is the form that brought itself into my life. The road has been a long and difficult one that has stretched out for more than one-third of my life. But, as each day, week, and year passes, the mileage between where I am today and my cancer experience gets greater and greater.

I was living what I believed to be the life of any average 19-year-old—going to college, but not entirely sure of what I wanted to be when I "grew up," and doing all of the usual things. I attended classes during the days and worked nights and weekends at a restaurant and a bar. I dated, but not seriously. So, things seemed to be what I would consider normal, until February 29, leap day, 1988.

The night before, I had been out late at a concert. So when I awoke with a ringing in my ears and feeling a little off balance, no alarms sounded. It was the difficulty seeing out of my right eye that sounded the first alarm, but I disregarded this because everything else was fine. I figured I must have slept wrong with a finger or something pressing on my eye. It would pass as the day went on, right? I went to class and noticed that my eye was not clearing up and that the unbalanced feeling was not getting any better. If anything, it was worse. At the end of class, I went to the college health center. The nurse there took one look in my eye and told me to go straight to the hospital. Upon my arrival at the hospital, the first of what would turn into thousands of blood tests was taken.

Within two hours of this initial blood test, I found myself in a Boston hospital surrounded by nurses, hematologists, ophthalmologists, and more different -ologists than one might think existed. The results of the initial blood test indicated that I was severely anemic with a hematocrit level of 11. The normal range is above 40. It was this, along with a low platelet count, that had caused my eye problem, a preretinal hemorrhage. In a bad-luck streak that had only just begun, this was the first break that I would catch; I could have just as easily suffered a cerebral hemorrhage that would have most certainly led to death. A further look into the blood tests would show the first signs of what caused the anemia—CML. I was hospitalized and received my first blood transfusion that same day.

I feel that I adapted to this news and the abrupt change in my life reasonably well, all things considered. As I saw it, there was nothing that I could have done to prevent it. It was not until I was in the hospital for a few days that I first got upset—angry, actually—and this was because I brushed my teeth and my gums bled. This was particularly upsetting to me because just a few hours prior, a nurse had told me that this would happen. Up until then, it had never happened.

The first hospitalization lasted 10 days, during which I received numerous transfusions and was started on a mild chemotherapeutic agent, which, taken daily by mouth, would ideally maintain the current state of my disease. I was released and allowed to go home. I returned to classes the next week but did stop working at that time, though. My schedule now included weekly trips to Boston to have my blood counts and general health checked. Usually, every two to three weeks the anemia would get the best of me, and I would require more blood transfusions. This schedule continued for several months, and as the summer came and classes ended, I returned to work in a somewhat limited capacity. On several occasions, I required hospitalization for infections or other ailments related to the CML, such as gout, high fever, and reactions to antibiotics given to combat the very same fevers. These episodes were above and beyond the daily battle of trying to keep focused and strong. The mental battles were sometimes as hard, if not harder, to deal with.

I could have stayed with this regimen of chemotherapy and transfusions, but for how long? The present state of my leukemia might have been controlled by these measures alone, but it also easily could have progressed into an acute stage.

Although relatively new and not in widespread use, bone marrow transplant did offer some hope of a cure. The search began for a donor. The marrow I needed had to come from someone of the same or extremely similar genetic type, so members of my immediate family were tested first. My only brother was a high match, but the doctors were certain they could find better. As they got further from the source of my own genes, the chance of a match decreased. The next step was to search for an unrelated donor. Statistics say that there should be two people out of every 20,000 that have very similar genetic coding, but because everyone's type is not known, the odds are significantly worse. A search in the national and international donor banks was then initiated.

In 1988, bone marrow transplants from people who are not related to the patient were still experimental and were being performed only in Seattle, London, and Milwaukee. I went to Milwaukee, the closest of the three sites, to be evaluated as a potential candidate for a transplant. At only 20 years old, this was something I knew I had to do to live.

In the fall of 1988, I returned to school for a week, but it became too much to deal with, so I took time off. There were so many more important things to attend to. I was working a little and trying to maintain a relatively active life. I did not think that I looked ill—a little pale because of the anemia but generally normal-looking. I was attempting to continue dating during this time, as the need for companionship was definitely there. Some people would choose not to continue a relationship with me once they found out about my illness, while others were not bothered by my illness. When people shied away because of the illness, I could not blame them. Even I recognized the risk of getting involved when there was so much uncertainty, not to mention the personal risk of emotional vulnerability. I had, by this point, accepted the possibility of death, but I most definitely would be doing everything that I could to postpone that day. I continued my daily routine as usual, allowing as little interference as I could. My good friends and family stuck by me through all of the tough decisions and tough times. They helped me to try to maintain a normal life.

It was late January 1989 when a potential donor was found, and I was scheduled to go to the Milwaukee transplant unit in the middle of March. After almost a year of waiting, searching, and coping with leukemia, things had really begun to move now. As part of the preparation for the transplant, my spleen was removed. This was the first time that I had ever had any type of surgery. The spleen is normally the size of an average man's fist, but mine was the size of a football. The next step was to move to Milwaukee in March for additional testing and the transplant itself. All of the testing went smoothly, and I was admitted on March 13, my 21st birthday, to begin the actual transplant process.

I was prepared to spend at least six weeks in the hospital. I had some idea of what was in store for me, but no amount of information could truly have prepared me for what lay ahead. I had been told that the radiation and chemotherapy treatments that were needed to destroy the diseased marrow could be fatal themselves but that they were necessary for the transplant. I knew that, at the very least, they would make me ill and almost certainly cause me to lose my hair. Because I wanted to fight on my own terms, the day before I was admitted I had my father give me a mohawk haircut. So, there I was, with a weird haircut, some pictures of friends, and a collection of music to occupy my time, ready to move into a room where I would spend the next several weeks. I tried to get acclimated to my new surroundings. Just four hours later, I was told that there was a problem with the donor and there would be about a month's delay before they could think about starting the treatment again. This news was certainly a setback, but I was most disturbed by the fact that I had to go out in public with this mohawk.

I returned home, but the month went by quickly. Before I knew it, I was back in Milwaukee, ready to try again. The first three weeks of radiation, chemotherapy, and the actual infusion of new marrow are a narcotic blur, and some things probably are best forgotten. During this cloudy period, I had several hallucinations caused by the drugs. The only one that I really remember was when I saw two men outside the window of my room. These two men, one white and the other black, with white hair and beards, were both wearing white robes, swearing at me, and calling me to come out. This especially drew the nurses' attention because my room was on the eighth floor. This is the most memorable to me because I am convinced that one or both of these men were death coming to take me. There were other hallucinations, some much more comical, that were relayed to me by my nurses once the haze cleared.

The next six weeks were not easy ones. I was kept in an air-purified isolation room until the new marrow grafted and my white blood cell count began to rise. My parents took turns coming to Milwaukee to be with me, and several of my friends made the trip, as well. The staff members who treated me were supportive and friendly. Also, the mail I received from my brother and my friends back east truly helped to ease the isolation.

When I was younger, I read a book titled *Eric,* by Doris Lund. This book made an impact on me for reasons that I did not understand until I was diagnosed with leukemia. *Eric,* written by the boy's mother, is about a boy's battle with leukemia. In this book, Eric did everything he could and everything that he was told to do to fight the disease, but he did it on his own terms and remained as much in control of the situation as he could. I took this route, also, doing what I had to do to fight, but by my own rules.

During these weeks of hospital isolation, I tried to carry on with my life. I would sleep the mornings away and watch television late into the evening. The doctors had an idea that the patients should get up early, shower first thing, and get to sleep early. I eventually persuaded them that I would be making my own schedule.

The time eventually did pass, and the next step was to move from isolation to an apartment near the hospital until I reached 100 days post-transplant. After the 100 days, my doctor would feel confident that I was over the most immediate major hurdles and that I could then be supervised under the care of my regular doctor. This freedom lasted only a week because I developed an infection that put me back into the hospital. This happened in the end of May, and I remained in the hospital for another eight weeks, until the end of July.

This was a major setback for me, and depression set in, which actually may have contributed to the infections. The mind is so powerful. The social workers and staff in the BMT unit encouraged me to maintain positive thoughts, but it took a while to get back on track. The staff members who cared for me during the previous six weeks were still there, and that familiarity certainly helped. I had several different infections during this eight-week hospital stay. My spirits were deflated, but I continued to keep an eye on my goal to get back east before my friends returned to college for the new school year.

I did return east the second week of August. I left Milwaukee a little sooner than the doctors liked, but I persuaded them to give in. My doctors in Milwaukee coordinated my care with the doctors in Boston. Arrangements also were made for me to return to Milwaukee in a month for a checkup.

When I returned home, I still needed to be careful about the things I ate or came into contact with. Also, I still was taking up to 20 pills a day for various reasons. I was supposed to stay away from my dog and other animals because of the numerous germs they carry, but that was one thing that I would not do because of my attachment to her. Although I was tired and weak from all that I had been through, I still spent time with my friends as often as I could while they were around.

Life began to get somewhat smoother. My trips to Milwaukee became fewer and further apart, and my overall dependence on medical support lessened. The following March I turned 22, returned to work at my part-time job, and returned to college to complete my degree. Over the next few years, I still was followed by doctors in Boston and did require hospitalization several times. The hospitalizations were not directly related to the underlying CML but more to the strain and shock put on the body by the transplant and some of the drugs associated with it.

In the summer of 1992, I took part in the National Kidney Foundation's U.S. Transplant Games at the University of California, Los Angeles. Anyone who has had a lifesaving transplant is invited to participate. The games are arranged to bring patients together to share their stories and experiences with each other as well as to raise awareness for organ donor participation. I went as a member of Team Wisconsin, and although I did not win any medals, it was a positive and uplifting experience. It was a reassurance that I was not alone.

To the best of my knowledge, I was the 279th person to undergo a bone marrow transplant from an unrelated donor. To this day, I am told by doctors that I am doing better than most and that few, if any, are further out of transplant than me.

No one can say for sure what the future holds for me—medically or otherwise. The transplant was a possible cure, and so far, it appears to be just that. I do, however, worry every time something medically bothers me, and even though the doctors do not attribute it to CML or the transplant, I cannot help but to do just that. I am doing very well, almost what would be considered normal.

Amanda Dolezal

Type of cancer: Burkitt's lymphoma
Age at diagnosis: 15
Current age: 16
Occupation: Student

Amanda's advice: You need to know and believe that you will survive this horrible disease. It only will take control of your life if you let it. Just remember one thing—after you are cured, you have your whole life in front of you. Don't give up on any of your dreams.

Amanda's Cancer Journey

I was diagnosed with Burkitt's lymphoma in September 1997. It all started on the second day of my sophomore year of high school. I was sitting at lunch with some of my friends when my best friend asked me about the huge lump on the side of my neck. I didn't know what she was talking about, and I made her come to the bathroom with me. When I looked in the mirror, I couldn't believe it. Nothing had been there that morning. The lump seemed to appear in a matter of minutes.

I went home after school that day, but I wasn't worried about the lump. I told my mom, and we made a doctor's appointment for the following week. My family doctor told me it was possibly an abscessed tooth or a swollen lymph gland. He put me on some medication and told me to come back in a week if the lump hadn't gone down. After a week was up, the lump still looked exactly the same. My family doctor then referred me to an ear, nose, and throat specialist.

When I got to the specialist's office, he took a look at the lump and said that it might be a cyst. He then did a needle biopsy. In this procedure, three different needles were placed into the lump to draw out some tissue for a sample. After he drew out the tissue, he told me it was definitely not a cyst.

He told me it could be a tumor of some sort. That was when I swear my heart stopped. I was so frightened. The words *tumor* and *cancer* had never crossed my mind. There was absolutely no way this was happening to me, I thought.

The specialist sent the tissue samples to the Mayo Clinic. About three days later, the doctor called to tell my parents that I had Burkitt's lymphoma, a very fast-growing cancer. When I was told that I had cancer, I started sobbing hysterically. I thought I was going to die. My parents explained everything to me, but I still didn't think I was going to make it.

I was sent to Methodist Hospital in Indianapolis, IN, where I received my first chemotherapy treatments. I went through two cycles of chemotherapy. I stayed at Methodist for four days, and after that, I got the rest of my treatments at a hospital about a half an hour from my home.

I started losing my hair after three weeks of treatment. I would just lay on the couch every day. I couldn't eat or sleep. The chemo did a number on my stomach, and I lost about 20 pounds. I couldn't go outside because my blood cell counts were so low that the doctors were afraid I would get an infection. Even with the precautions, I did develop a very severe infection, anyway. As a result, my parents were taught, at home, how to hook my IVs up to a catheter that was implanted in my chest. I was on medication for a week, and finally the infection cleared up.

After my two cycles of chemotherapy were over, my blood cell count was 1.0, which is very dangerous. I had to have two blood transfusions.

I've been in remission for seven months, and the doctors say that, after two years of remission, I will be considered cured.

Samuel Robert Frost

Type of cancer: Testicular cancer
Age at diagnosis: 17
Current age: 35
Occupation: Systems analyst
Sam's advice: Cancer is beatable. It is not a death sentence, but beating it won't be easy. Accommodate your doctors and treatment schedule, but don't give up your life. Get involved in the decision-making process because this will help you to stay in control. Do as much as you can.

Sam's Cancer Journey

I am the youngest of three children. My mom is a school teacher, and my dad is a minister. Although we moved around a lot when I was growing up, my family never really moved that far. Basically, I am a Pennsylvania boy who routinely gets accused of having an Irish temper and a Pennsylvania Dutch stubbornness.

I played football and volleyball and wrestled in high school. I played baseball, basketball, and tennis at the recreation league level. I also played the piano, violin, and electric bass and sang in the church choir. I was president of the National Honor Society and voted Most Likely to Succeed. I generally was convinced that I was immortal and one of the greatest guys to walk the face of the earth.

Then, while undergoing a physical to gain my appointment to the United States Air Force Academy, the doctor took about 30 minutes to do the dreaded "cough" test, which made me wonder what on earth he was doing. The thought of something being wrong with me never entered my mind. The Army doctor told me to get my parents. They then dismissed me; 10 minutes later, Pop came out of the office and said that we were going to Hershey Medical Center. Pop said that the Army doc wanted some tests done and that it was no big deal. We made the 20-minute drive in silence. I figured this beat the heck out of sitting in school.

Upon arriving at Hershey, we parked and strolled down to the family practice clinic because my dad knew some of the doctors. While they talked, I started looking for the urology clinic. I found it, went back, and got my dad, and we walked down there for my appointment. I had a 2:30 pm appointment. It's amazing how that sticks out in my mind because half of the time I can't remember what day it is. The nurse did the standard checks: blood pressure, pulse, breathing, weight, and height. Then I went in to see the doctor. The doctor told me to "drop my drawers" and in three nanoseconds made a diagnosis; he told me that I had cancer and needed to be admitted to the hospital right away. Needless to say, I handled this information like any mature 17-year-old would—I started to cry and said that I wanted my dad.

The Journey Begins: I was diagnosed with cancer when I was a senior in high school. I checked into the hospital early Monday morning. I don't remember much of that day except for passing out on this teeny-tiny nurse who took my blood. Later that night, I was watching the Rams on Monday Night Football®, and the nurses kept coming in to check on me, wondering why I hadn't fallen asleep. Looking back on this, I'm still struck by the unreality of it all; I was 17, in great shape, and sitting in bed waiting to get cut. No one told me what would happen if it was malignant; no one told me what would happen if it was benign; no one told me anything except, "It'll be okay. You'll be fine." I'm not sure what I wanted to know because I am damn sure that I would not have been calm, composed, or anything else if someone would have told me that they were going to cut off one of my testicles.

The surgery came and went. I vaguely recall being told that it was cancerous, but they had removed the tumor and everything was going to be fine because testicular cancer is very curable. It was on Wednesday when I realized that my life had definitely changed. That's when I discovered that removing the tumor included removing the testicle, and the cure was going to include four months of chemotherapy. First, I needed to have a few tests to determine if the cancer had spread. I wasn't exactly ecstatic about this information, but everyone was upbeat and all parts of my body seemed to be working, so I thought, Why cry about it?

Then came the chemotherapy. My parents and oncologist decided that the less time I spent in the hospital, the better. So, I did my chemotherapy as an outpatient. I had four cycles of bleomycin, vinblastine, and cisplatinum. Every three weeks, I had to stay in the hospital. I would arrive before 7 am, get an IV started, and, over the course of the day, receive the cisplatinum, which would make me extremely nauseous—think projectile vomiting. I'd stay in Hershey's ambulatory care area overnight, puking my guts out and thinking, Why me? The next day, the sun would come up, and it would be over for another three weeks.

I still hadn't told the people at school that I had cancer. Somehow, it was hard to work it into the flow of conversation with my guy friends. "Hey, she is kinda cute! Did I tell you that I only have one testicle?" It was definitely not a topic I'd bring up on a date. Gradually, as I got done with the tests and the first cycle of chemotherapy, people started asking why I was absent so often, and then I began to tell.

The next trial I endured was losing my hair. It was a cold January day, and I was at the playground playing basketball with a bunch of kids from high school. We were wearing sweats and knit hats, and a couple of girls were watching. In a moment of temporary insanity, I flew down the lane for a finger-roll lay-up. Someone hacked me with a forearm to the head. I called "ball" and noticed that everyone was staring at me. I remained calm, cool, and collected and started to claim that, of course, it's a foul and wondered what was the matter. My friend walked up, picked my hat off of the ground, leaned toward me, and said that I was bald. Looking at my hat, I saw that he was right because it was filled with hair. After we finished the game, I went home, took a shower, and looked in the mirror. At that moment, I wasn't bald. It was worse. I had hair on part of my head and was bald in other spots. I actually looked like I was sick or something.

After consulting with two of my friends, I made the decision to shave my head. Now, looking like "Mr. Clean" in front of my family and two really good friends was one thing, but going out in public was another. My two friends took charge by escorting me to the Sunny Surplus in York, PA. They recommended hats, and I tried on about a million of them. We picked out an olive green United States Marine Corps PFC hat that cost me something like $2. So, $2 poorer but a hat richer, we left. I pretty much wore that hat for the next five months, and it was one of the best investments I ever made.

High school passed, and so did the cancer treatments. While continuing my monthly checkups at Hershey, I would be sweating bullets and snapping at everyone the day before and the day of. I'm a big chicken who hates needles, passing out if I ever am dumb enough to look at them drawing my blood. After a couple of months, I started thinking that I had beaten cancer. Sure, I had a few scars from surgery and a few more long, dark-brown lines from chemotherapy, and my hair was short but growing, but I thought that I had done it—I had beaten cancer.

Then came one of the most memorable moments in my life. At one of my checkups, my doctor said that I had a lump on the other testicle and he wanted me to come back into the hospital for the same stuff that they had done a year or so ago. Again, I handled it the way any mature 19-year-old guy would: I cussed out the doctor and told him there was no way I was going through that again. I got two other opinions, but both physicians recommended surgery. Both also suggested that if I ever wanted a chance at having my own children, I should make a deposit in a sperm bank.

The trip to New York to go to the sperm bank was cool. I had only been to New York once before, and although I was really nervous about going to a sperm bank, I was excited about going to the top of the Empire State Building, walking around Central Park, and seeing the Statue of Liberty. I had this picture of the sperm bank being this huge laboratory with doctors, nurses, and needles. And how were they going to get the sperm out of me? Well, for those of you who are as naive as I was, there is no laboratory and no doctors and nurses—just a bunch of small rooms with easy chairs and couches and piles of men's magazines and the receptionist hands you a plastic cup.

The Journey Continues: I chose the doctors in Baltimore at Johns Hopkins Hospital because I was going to school at Western Maryland College. I didn't have a good feeling about the upcoming surgery. My then-girlfriend and now wife, Jackie, called my fraternity brothers, and they came to visit me. The surgery went without a hitch, but the pathology report came back with the word *malignant*. After a discussion with my oncologist about my bad attitude, we decided that surveillance was the best way to go.

The surveillance lasted for six months, but tests indicated that I needed more chemotherapy. I swore at the end of the first go-around with chemotherapy that I would die before I did it again. My oncologist recommended seeing a psychiatrist to try to help me to get through it again. I went, but for whatever reason, it didn't really help. I could do amazing things with my pulse rate, blood pressure, and body temperature as long as I was in the psychiatrist's office, but put me back in the treatment room and I was a raving lunatic. I pulled the IV out a couple of times. I went through two cycles of the recommended four. My oncologist let it slip that the chemotherapy was not working, and I got up and walked out of the treatment room.

Time-Out: When I walked out of the treatment room in March 1983, I was done with cancer, chemotherapy, and everyone in the medical profession. What had they done for me? I had no testicles. I only continued to act like a man because I was taking anabolic steroids. I also was bald again. I had been cut by the baseball team, partially because of a lack of talent, but partially because of the coach's inability to handle me going through chemotherapy. I had no responsibilities. I enjoyed the heck out of that semester of college. I went back home that summer and I worked, played softball, saw my girlfriend, went to a bunch of concerts, and just had a great time loving life and doing what I wanted to do. Life was good. I blew off checkups for that whole summer but promised my mom and girlfriend that I'd go once school started.

The Journey Resumed: With school starting, fall baseball started pretty quickly. I had quit playing football because I looked in the mirror and realized that my best days were behind me. I also had dislocated my right shoulder during wrestling season the year before and just had no desire to play anymore. While playing baseball, my back started to hurt, and I just assumed that I had pulled a muscle. Honestly, I didn't even think that the cancer had come back.

I was going to my check-ups again, but I didn't tell anyone my back was hurting. Some of my tests came back suspicious, and I had more tests. A CT scan revealed enlarged lymph nodes, and I was told that, if I wanted to survive, I needed to have surgery followed by chemotherapy. Period. Case closed. I walked out of the office repeating my previous vow. My family and friends started turning on the guilt machine, but I held them off for a while. Now, 15 years later, I still don't know how they talked me into it, but they did, and I'm glad.

The surgery is something called retroperitoneal lymph node dissection (RPLND). Nowadays, they talk about "nerve-sparing" RPLND. They told me that there was a good chance that I would lose the ability to have sex. I was 20 years old and they were telling me the cheery news that this surgery had a good chance of rendering me impotent. Fortunately, it didn't.

The surgery was nasty. I have a 10-inch scar running from the bottom of my sternum to my waist. I had a tube in my nose, a catheter, an IV running right into my neck, and probably other horrible stuff that I blocked out of my mind. My oncologist recommended immediate chemotherapy, but because he is such a good guy, he let me talk him into letting me play baseball that spring. I made the team, and either I got incredibly more talented in a year, or the coach got a lot more sympathetic. Whatever happened, we won our conference and were ranked nationally for a while. Even knowing that I had chemotherapy coming up that summer, I still had a great semester.

In the summer of 1984, I was admitted to Johns Hopkins. My doctor wasn't playing around this time; he ordered that I receive a Hickman™ catheter because I was such a big baby when it came to needles and IVs. A Hickman catheter is a tube that is surgically placed directly into the brachial vein. From the catheter, two clear plastic tubes run out through a person's chest. These tubes must be rinsed daily with saline and heparin solution, and they can't get wet. No showers or swimming for me. Anyway, the Hickman was inserted, and the next day, chemotherapy was started again. This time, I underwent chemotherapy as an inpatient. I had one of the greatest oncology nurses. I stayed in the hospital for five days and received chemotherapy through my Hickman. They also took blood through the Hickman so that I wouldn't have to get stuck with needles.

After five days, I went home and started working and playing softball again. Things went well for two weeks, and then I went back to the hospital to do it again. Things continued to go well, and, although the chemotherapy wasn't fun, I didn't have to go through daily fights to find a good vein or have a vein collapse during treatment so that the nurse had to find another one. This made things better than they were.

So I went home again to my normal routine, feeling happy because everything looked to be progressing nicely. Then, during one game soon after my second treatment, I was going from first to third on a single, and since it was a close play, I slid in. I got a heck of a "strawberry" and kept playing.

The next day, I went to work even though I didn't feel good. I worked for an ice company doing manual labor in a 40° warehouse, and I was sweating like a pig. Without my knowledge, my boss and coworkers called my parents, who called the hospital. With a temperature of 105°, I was rushed to Johns Hopkins. They doctors knew I had a raging infection, but they didn't know why. I had so many tests that I don't even remember what they all were.

After a day of tests, my favorite oncology nurse noticed that I was limping and asked me why. I showed her my "strawberry." That was the source of my infection. My white blood cell levels were so low that I stayed in the hospital. I was given some type of drug to stimulate white blood cell production. My doctor wasn't happy because he felt that, if the timing were off on my chemotherapy, it's effectiveness would decrease. I was in the hospital for the rest of the summer. Well, I did get out for a few Orioles baseball games.

The Journey Ends?: In August of 1984, my chemotherapy ended. All of my test results came back negative. My lungs are scarred, but they will always be. And, my hair was growing in for a third time. My doctor was happy, my family and friends were happy, and I was playing fall baseball again. I eventually graduated from college, married Jackie, got a job, and started graduate school. We also started a family.

No one knows that I had cancer until I tell them. I'm not sure why I got it in the first place, and I sure as heck don't know why I survived, but I did. I believe in God and a divine plan. He doesn't give us anything we can't handle without His help. I also look for humor and wisdom everywhere.

Kimberley Hagood

Type of cancer: Lymphoma
Age at diagnosis: 14
Current age: 16
Occupation: Student
Kimberley's advice: This will be hard. I'm not going to lie about that. No matter what happens, you can't give up. Fight hard, be strong, and see what comes out of it. You can do it.

Kimberley's Cancer Journey

On December 6, 1995, at the age of 14, I was diagnosed with large cell histiocytic non-Hodgkin's lymphoma, a very aggressive cancer.

About six months before I was diagnosed, I lost a lot of weight. I was 5'6" and 75 lbs. My family noticed laziness, mood swings, and an overall personality change. My mom knew that something bad was happening to me, and she took me for medical help. One doctor decided that I was anorexic because of the weight loss and because I couldn't eat anything. My mom was not satisfied with that diagnosis.

She took me to doctors all over the place, and we were turned away with no answers. My mom kept trying. Finally, a doctor admitted me to the hospital for testing because, by this time, I had lost so much weight and was so weak that I couldn't hold myself up. I also had a large bump in my pelvis area. The doctors did several tests and eventually took a biopsy of the bump that had swollen up so much that it hurt to move.

It took a week for the results of the tests to come back. The doctors told my parents the news, and then my dad told me. I remember laughing at him, thinking it was some kind of joke. I soon realized that he wasn't kidding. I was scared and asked if I was going to die. There were no positive answers. At that moment, I looked over at my mom. She was pale and scared out of her mind. I decided that I had to try to be strong not only for myself but also for my family because the odds were strongly against me. After I decided that, I began to worry about losing my long, blond hair, which I did end up losing during my chemotherapy treatments. I wore baseball hats to cover my bald head until I became comfortable with the little stubs I had.

The day after I was told that I had cancer, I was scheduled to undergo surgery to have a catheter implanted in my chest. The doctors wanted to start chemotherapy right away. I had various chemotherapy experiences. Some of them were performed as outpatient procedures, and, for some, I had to stay in the hospital for three to four days. This lasted for a year and a half. I had the normal complications that went along with chemotherapy, such as vomiting and fevers, but overall it went well.

I kept up with my normal daily routine. I had played tennis for eight years before I was diagnosed with cancer and played as much as possible during the time I was in treatment. I played on the varsity high school tennis team for two years and had great seasons. I tried my hardest, and that was more than people asked of me.

All totaled, I had seven surgeries, chemotherapy, and five weeks of Monday-through-Friday radiation treatments. Finally, it was over. I was so scared, but my family and friends helped me through it. My mom was there for me all of the time, spending nights in the hospital with me. My dad made me laugh and brought me food. My younger sister stood up for me and made me forget that I was sick. If it wasn't for my family and friends, I probably would have given up, but they kept me fighting. I am so happy that they didn't let me give up because I won a battle with all of the odds stacked against me.

To my family and friends, you mean the world to me. I love you, guys.

Susan Johnston

Type of cancer: Synovial sarcoma
Age at diagnosis: 20
Current age: 24
Occupation: Sales representative
Susan's advice: Cancer isn't a death sentence, so don't let anyone treat you like it is. Do everything you want to do. It's your life—enjoy it to the fullest and learn to appreciate it.

Susan's Cancer Journey

So there I was, a happy college student, daydreaming about who I'd go out with that night as I waited for the results of my biopsy. I had a bump on the inside of my arm that wouldn't go away, and I was concerned because it was cutting off circulation in my hand. I never imagined that this thing would change my entire life. I still remember it like it was yesterday.

My dad and I waited for the doctor. From the sad look on my doctor's face, I knew it was bad. "This is a cancerous tumor," he said solemnly. My mouth dropped, and my heart nearly stopped. Every emotion known to man suddenly came out. At first, I didn't believe him. I thought he was an idiot. I knew I was healthy and didn't believe this was happening to me.

Soon, he began telling me the options that I had to work with. I wasn't paying any attention and tuned him out. I thought he was full of it. How dare he tell me this? He's so wrong. I then became very angry and disgusted. I didn't want to talk to anyone there.

I looked at my dad and saw the sadness on his face. I understood that this was serious, and that made me cry.

I was diagnosed with a rare cancer called synovial sarcoma. It affects the tissue next to the bone, the synovial sack. Because it is so rare, it is hard to detect. Knowing this didn't make me feel much better, just more alone.

I left the doctor's office, knowing that I had to get more tests to determine which road to take. I was scared more than I had ever been before. I was living in a dorm on campus and decided to go back to my room. I knew that if I went back home, seeing my mom would have been even more devastating. My dad urged me to come home, but I refused. I think a part of me really wanted to be alone to absorb all of this. My mom called me, crying, and I lost it, too. We were confused, scared, and lost and didn't know what to do or how to handle this.

As I sat there crying and talking to my mom, two of my friends came in my room. They were very understanding and felt for me. The first words out of one of my friend's mouth were, "Well, when you lose your hair, I can give you my leather coat and you can be a punk." Everyone's mouth dropped until they saw me laughing and smiling. I needed that reassurance. I needed to know that my friends would still love me and not look at me like a sick person. I think that also is the reason I called all of my friends that night and told them.

At my next doctor's appointment, I was to find out if the cancer had spread to my lungs. I sat up all night before the tests and thought about my whole life as if it were ending. This was the first real spiritual contact I had with God that I could remember.

As I sat there, thinking and crying, I felt an unbelievable weight being lifted from me. I felt as though someone was there with me, reassuring me that things were going to be okay. I could never explain the feeling to others. I guess I knew that was a feeling I had to hold on to. Sure enough, the tests came back clear.

I began my radiation treatments and also started dating. I remember being terrified of telling my date about my illness. I thought he'd be as disgusted by it as I was. Two days before I had surgery, he asked me to a fraternity formal. The surgery didn't seem so bad anymore.

When the day came for surgery, I was nervous, but not as nervous as I think I should have been. It lasted for five hours. They were taking out the tumor and determining if it was going to be necessary to amputate my arm. I had either forgotten about the fact that I might lose my arm, or I just knew everything was going to be okay. I had no fear. I believe God was with me.

When I awoke, my parents were waiting. I was thirsty and begged for anything to drink. They urged me not to, but I won—and ended up vomiting all over myself. I didn't seem to care. I laughed and figured I was alive and felt great considering the circumstances. And I still had two arms.

I stayed in the hospital for five days, and each day I felt better. Even though few people visited me, which hurt, I had the people I loved most by my side. The surgery had gone better than my doctors had anticipated.

I was so anxious to get home. My mom had to help me with everything, though. I don't know what I would have done without her.

After being cooped up for so long, I broke out and was encouraged by friends to go out and celebrate life. However, chemotherapy soon hit like a boulder. It knocked me hard on my butt. I felt so sick, and it really brought my spirits down. I had six sessions of outpatient treatment, and it seemed to last forever.

After my second treatment, I began to lose some hair. I decided to shave my head to avoid any embarrassing hassles. I was scared but just wanted to do it fast. As I was leaving my house, a friend called. I told him what I was doing and that I had to go. He volunteered to shave his head, too. Hearing this made me cry. I urged him not to, but it was nice to know that he would do something like that for me.

When I finally lost all of my hair, I wore a wig. It was hot, itchy, and uncomfortable, but I didn't want people to stare or ask questions. I showed some of my friends my bald look and got many different reactions. A few stared or looked away in horror, while others giggled. Soon, people got used to it and didn't care. They knew I was comfortable with it so they could be comfortable with it, too. However, I avoided public reaction to my bald head by always wearing my wig. One close friend of mine, who happens to be a beautician, had the best reaction. She looked at my head and said, "Wow, you have a really nicely shaped head, no bumps or anything." She would always rub my head and call me the cute little bald girl.

While I was receiving chemotherapy, I had to watch my white blood cell counts. I was prone to illnesses, which could set me back and postpone my chemotherapy. I had to stay away from crowds and avoid sick people. I chose one friend to hang out with during the times when my counts were low. She was always there to listen to me, and often we played Nintendo® into the early hours of the morning. Finally, the end of my chemo had arrived. I was completely hairless and utterly exhausted but overjoyed to get past it and move on with my life.

During the year that I was sick, I faced death and decided I wasn't done living yet. This was a smack in the face for me to wake up and enjoy each day because there may not be a next day. I also realized who my real friends were.

I went through a long stage of loneliness. Not only was my cancer rare, but I was young and also dealing with many other problems. Trying to find someone with my cancer and around my age was next to impossible. I needed to understand how others coped so that I could cope myself. Each day was a new challenge and a different fight.

The atmosphere around me became repetitive and annoying. I got tired of people asking, "How do you feel?" with that pathetic look on their faces. They didn't really want to hear my problems. I became tired of people using my disease as a way to get to talk about their own problems. I soon learned that people were either ignorant or confused. They didn't know how to treat me.

Five years later, I've realized how much I've learned. People still ask the familiar "How are you feeling?" question. I guess I've learned to smile and say, "Great. Glad you care."

People today stop and say, "Wow, you fought cancer and won." I realize that I didn't fight any harder than others. I believe that my time wasn't up yet. There are things I still need to do.

Adam Kabel

Type of cancer: Hodgkin's disease
Age at diagnosis: 15
Current age: 25
Occupation: Working on a career in aviation
Adam's advice: Aside from all of the standard advice such as "Never give up" and

"Don't let it get you down," I suggest keeping a diary of everything you went through or are going through. I didn't, but wish I had. Cancer isn't something you want to have, but it's something you'll never want to forget. Really. No joke.

Adam's Cancer Journey

I remember walking through a mall with my dad in mid-August of 1989. I was 15. My dad put his hand around my neck and felt a lump. Thinking it was nothing, but just to be sure, we told my mom and she set up an appointment with my doctor.

The doctor felt the lump and gave me antibiotics. He said it was probably just a swollen gland, a condition common in teenagers. That also was my first memory of getting a blood test. I hated it. I never wanted to have another one. So much for that wish.

I took the medicine, and after I had finished it, my mom and I went back to see the doctor. He felt the lump again, and the look on his face said it all. The lump hadn't shrunk but rather grew. He called the surgeon on his car phone and told us to meet him in the emergency room of the hospital.

In the emergency room, the surgeon felt the lump for about five minutes and said that he was 95% sure that it was malignant. I had a biopsy a few days later—my first surgery. They wanted to inject the anesthetic into me to put me to sleep, but I insisted on the gas. I hate needles. While I was asleep, the surgeon also performed a bone marrow biopsy and a spinal tap. At least I was asleep.

School was about to start, but that was the least of my worries. I remember my parents and some of their friends sitting around the house, waiting for the phone to ring. My mom answered it and turned to us. As tears rolled down her face, she said, "It's Hodgkin's."

After the initial diagnosis, I had a whole bunch of scans and tests performed to see the extent of the cancer. I remember one of the scans for which I had to lay perfectly still for 45 minutes with my arms over my head while this big thing slowly rotated around me. That hurt.

I had my spleen and appendix removed about two weeks after the initial diagnosis, as well as many biopsies of my internal lymph nodes.

I spent my 16th birthday in the hospital recovering from the surgery. In the end, I was diagnosed with stage IIIA. I had cancer cells in my neck, throat, abdomen, and spleen.

By the way, I missed school for the month of September and had tutors during that time. Well, at least some good came out of this. If I got sick of school work, I could always say I was getting tired. Hey, whatever works.

After the weeks of surgery and tests, it was time to start treatment. I was to have 12 treatments of combination chemotherapy followed by radiation therapy. I received the chemotherapy every other Friday.

I had a central line put in at the end of September 1989, and it remained in place for about a year. Although I was scheduled to have it put in at noon, I didn't actually have the surgery until around 7 pm. I wasn't allowed to eat that whole day.

As if that wasn't enough, I had my first chemo treatment that same night. The chemo made me so sick that I ended up spending the night in the hospital.

I missed school to go to my next chemotherapy session. First, I had to have a blood test. I found out that my blood counts were too low to receive the treatment, so I went back to school for the rest of the day. That turned out to be one of the happiest days of my life. I was thrilled.

The next Friday, though, my blood counts were fine. Chemo, which we didn't know at the time, turned out to be an all-day event. One of my parents went with me to the treatment clinic, and sometimes the other would meet up with us later in the day.

We'd get to the clinic around 10 am. I'd have a blood test done, and if my counts were high enough, I would have an IV hooked up to my central line, and treatment would begin. Ironically, I was so nervous that I'd start throwing up around 11 am while the antinausea medication was going in.

It took about two hours to administer the four chemo drugs, and I'd be puking constantly. At around 4 or 5 pm, we'd head home. We timed it for right after I threw up. It's a good thing that we only lived a couple of minutes from where I had the treatments. As soon as I got home, I'd run into the house and upstairs to the bathroom. I would be sick until I fell asleep that evening around 11 or midnight. I hated Fridays.

After I fell asleep on Friday night, I woke up on Saturday like nothing had happened. I wasn't sick or anything. I even went to the mall one Saturday after having received chemo treatment on Friday. However, on Sunday I felt sick again. I stayed home from school to recover on Monday and sometimes on Tuesday. I usually wound up missing at least one day of school a week, unless my blood counts were low; then, I'd only miss half a day.

This went on for about eight months. It came to a point when, instead of living day to day, my family and I lived from chemo to chemo. My parents would schedule their work around the chemo Fridays so they could go with me. On what was supposed to be my last treatment, something happened and the IV needle slipped out slightly. We didn't notice it until we looked on the floor and saw the red drug leaking out. I had to go back again to receive the rest of the drug.

I then had radiation therapy, which was a party compared to chemo. I got sick the first time, but antinausea pills stopped that. Almost a year after diagnosis, I was finished with all of my treatments.

I lost most of my hair, but I never wore a wig. My dad and I went looking for one, but I really didn't want to wear one, so I always wore a Cubs hat.

While visiting my grandparents in England, I developed shingles. I was in major pain on the plane ride home and then spent a week in the hospital. I had a bit of fun in the hospital, though. The medicine I had to take for shingles was given through an IV. After one of the IV bags was empty, my mom took it down, slit the top open, cleaned it, and filled it with water. She then went to the pet shop, got a goldfish, put it in the bag, and taped the IV line to me so it looked like it was going into me.

Doctors and nurses from the entire hospital were called in to take a look at this new treatment. I also liked to mess around with the electronic IV drip. After a nurse set it up, I'd make it start beeping, so she'd have to keep coming in and fixing it. She eventually caught on.

The Starlight Foundation gave my family and me a free cruise in the midst of my treatment. They arranged for a limo to pick us up at our house and flew us to Miami. We stayed overnight in a hotel and then embarked on a seven-day cruise. Those guys did a great job.

I'm now 24 and a graduate of Embry-Riddle Aeronautical University in Daytona Beach, FL.

Jim Keefe

Type of cancer: Hodgkin's disease
Age at diagnosis: 19
Current age: 38
Occupation: Teacher
Jim's advice: Keep a positive attitude and have faith that the cancer will be cured. Cancer is no longer a death sentence. It is only a speed bump on the road of life.

Jim's Cancer Journey

I was diagnosed with Hodgkin's disease on December 11, 1979, at the age of 19. My Hodgkin's disease started as a big lump in my neck, on the right side. My doctor thought it was probably a cyst. I was not too concerned about it because I had lumps in my neck and on the back of my neck before, most of them caused by acne. This lump was the size of my fist. The doctor performed a biopsy and removed the lump on December 5, 1979.

After it was determined that the lump was cancerous, I had several tests to determine the stage of my Hodgkin's disease. The tests showed that I was in stage IVA. I did not need, or get, a splenectomy, which was rare 18 years ago, as the removal of the spleen was very common in the staging process.

Over six months, I underwent six cycles of chemotherapy. Tests results indicated that while the first six-month cycle of chemotherapy made major progress in the treatment of the cancer, it had not completed the job. I then received another six months of treatment.

In December 1980, just two weeks before my 21st birthday, I finished my last treatment. I returned to college the following January. I had checkups every three months for a year, then every four months for a year, and then every six months for a year. I now see my regular family doctor to have a chest x-ray usually every two years. I don't really think about having them done anymore, and the doctors don't either—not 18 years after my diagnosis.

I have told many people that my cancer experience forced me to grow up and mature fast. I was 19 when I was diagnosed, spent all of my 20th year on chemotherapy, and could not even go out for my first legal drink of alcohol on my 21st

birthday because I had just completed my chemotherapy treatment. I did have one hell of a private celebration, though. I was given a guarded, but clean, bill of health and a second chance at life.

I want everyone to know that cancer can be beaten and that there is light at the end of the tunnel. I am living proof.

Jennifer McFerrin

Type of cancer: Choriocarcinoma and anaplastic astrocytoma
Age at diagnosis: 7 (with choriocarcinoma) and 17 (with anaplastic astrocytoma)
Current age: 22
Status: Still recovering
Jennifer's advice: Trust in God and look to your family for support.

Jennifer's Cancer Journey

I was diagnosed with my first brain tumor, a choriocarcinoma, when I was seven years old. After two surgeries, radiation, and two-and-one-half years of chemotherapy, we thought I was free of cancer.

Ten years later, I was diagnosed with my second brain tumor, an anaplastic astrocytoma, which doctors believed may have been related to the radiation therapy used to cure the first tumor. Because my second tumor was located in the optic chiasm, my doctors did not want to operate. However, my mom found a neurosurgeon at New York University Hospital who had expertise in this area. The surgery did not go as well as we had hoped. I had a stroke during surgery and a severe reaction to the drug phenytoin, which kept me in intensive care for three weeks. The doctor was unable to remove all of the tumor.

After six weeks of healing, I started on a chemotherapy regimen at M.D. Anderson Cancer Center in Houston, TX. Following six weeks of chemotherapy, my immune system became so depressed that I developed a herpes zoster infection (shingles), which went into my brain and put me in a coma for 10 days. The coma brought back the weakness of the first stroke, which left me unable to talk or even swallow. However, after speech therapy, physical therapy, and occupational therapy, I am doing much better.

Today, I am still fighting my way back from the cancer and the problems caused by the many treatments. I feel that each year provides new research and treatments, which gives me hope that I will one day be cancer-free.

Christine Mizen

Type of cancer: Hodgkin's disease
Age at diagnosis: 17
Current age: 27
Occupation: Nanny, student
Christine's advice: When you get to the end of your rope, tie a knot and hold on.

Christine's Cancer Journey

Sometimes, I wonder if it really happened to me. I remember thinking this before, when I was going through it. Now, I have the scars that are always there to remind me. When I look at them, I know it did happen.

I was diagnosed with Hodgkin's disease when I was 17 years old and about to start my senior year of high school. At this point in my young life, I was convinced that life was a crock. I was miserable. I could never see past tomorrow. I was the epitome of angst-ridden youth. Emotionally, I felt like a goober, and physically, like a 70-year-old. Sure, I had some fun times, but deep inside I knew there was something wrong with me. I was always so cold and tired. I had this biology teacher who let me sit on the heater in his classroom. I would lean up against the window, as my butt was burning off, trying to maintain a look of interest so I would not anger the teacher and lose my position of warmth.

I can recall looking in the bathroom mirror before class, acknowledging this huge lump on my throat, and yet still shrugging it off. Nothing could have possibly been wrong with me. I was a teenager. I was more concerned with my hair. I was either cutting it off or growing it in. I believed that it didn't matter what your face was like because your hair could redeem you. I was always so tired that I would stay in bed for an extra few minutes. Those minutes were heaven, but I always left time to fix my hair. As I have said, it had been the most important aspect of my shallow youth.

Finally, a guy from my brother's fraternity house told me that I really should get my lump checked out. It had grown larger and was very noticeable. I was still ignoring it, thinking it would go away. Guess what? It didn't. I ended up with a diagnosis of goiter, an enlargement of my thyroid. I was treated with thyroid medicine for a year before I sought a second opinion. I am so glad I did.

I will never forget the day I was diagnosed with Hodgkin's disease. I went to my doctor's office to hear the results of the zillions of tests I had been through. I sat in the office waiting for more than two hours. My doctor was running late but did not want me to reschedule. This would have clued anyone else in, but of course, I was not anyone else. I was reading a magazine. When the doctor arrived, he sat down and said, "Kiddo, you have cancer." The word echoed in my head, and I just sat there trying to register what he had just said. When it finally registered, I nearly wet my pants. Suddenly, I snapped out of my daze. I don't know where I found the strength, but I did. "Okay," I said. "What do I have to do?"

I left the office in a numb, tough-girl mode and went straight to Taco Bell™, the video store, and the gas station. I picked up a load of junk food, George Carlin videos, and two packs of cigarettes. Hey, if this was how it was going to be, I might as well live it up.

The first treatment was terrifying. I had no idea what to expect. No one had let me in on any of the secrets. I had browsed through a book on chemotherapy, but for the most part, I was on my own. After the first week, my golden locks were still there. I thought that, maybe, I was one of those lucky people you hear of who don't lose their hair. I knew that I might lose my hair later on, so I went out and bought some outrageous red hair dye. I was rebelling in any way I could. Of course, the dye job did not work because of all the chemicals in the therapy. I had wasted my money and any hopes of being a redhead.

I received chemotherapy treatments every other week. After a couple of rounds, my hair started to get rubbery. The texture was like spongy plastic. Every time I washed it or brushed it, bits of hair would fall out. After a while, I stopped messing with it. I needed my crowning glory for all it was worth, but I ended up looking like Pig Pen from the Charlie Brown cartoon.

About this same time, I developed a blood clot in my heart. This was dangerous stuff. The clot was the size of a golf ball, and it was moving back and forth, waiting to drop and get caught in a valve of my heart. When it was detected, I was admitted to the intensive-care unit in the hospital. I had left the house without my magazines or books, so I was bored out of my skin. Everyone in the unit was in a coma, and the nurses were no fun at all. I tried to be as sweet as my teen years would allow and begged for a television. I won them over, but of course, they had forgotten the remote, and you know how high those televisions are in the hospital. I was constantly being monitored and was not allowed to move, let alone get up to use the bathroom. I don't know about you, but this was a huge dilemma for me. I swore I would hold it until I was set free, for there was no way that this tough girl was going to use a bed pan.

Under these circumstances, and with the channel of my wondrous television set on some idiotic show, I was just not in the mood to deal with anyone. I had just had an argument with this stupid doctor who knew nothing about how to deal with an obnoxious youth. He had insisted on poking at my veins to no avail. By this time, I felt like an old pro at this cancer stuff. I kept telling him to let me have a hot rag to put on my veins to help the blood flow. Then, instead of all the pain he was giving me, he would get a good vein into which he could inject whatever he wanted. After many failed attempts, he finally listened to me. I didn't forget this, especially when he had the honor of giving me a rectal exam to check for internal bleeding. If you think that I made this easy for him, then you haven't figured me out yet!

So, there I was, with IVs in both arms, watching this stupid show on the tube. After all that had transpired this night, I was not about to take this inhumanity. What was I supposed to do, lay there and look at the ceiling and contemplate my life? I think not. I decided to get creative. I scooted to the edge of my bed and turned the channels with my big toe. Every time I did this, I would flash the nurses' station right across my glass bubble of a room. I was not wearing panties under my gown. Do you know how hard it is to pick a wedgie with both of your arms filled with IVs? I reveled in the outside shock every time I changed the channel.

For the most part, my family did not know how to handle me. My brothers were the worst. They really had a hard time watching their baby sister endure this horrible mess, and this blood clot sent them into a panic. They basically avoided me but knew they had to visit me in the intensive-care unit. The best part of all this drama was when my brother came to see me. It was my second day in the unit, and

I was not in my most pleasant frame of mind. By this time, I had decided to call a truce with the bedpan. Every time I got up the courage to use the pan, at least five doctors would waltz into my room, clipboards in hand. Whenever this happened, I got the inevitable stage fright. There I was—up to my eyeballs in it and not a single person to tangle with.

My brother came into the room, looking like he could bolt at any moment. He sat down in a chair facing me and tried not to look at my sparse head of hair. I tried to make him feel more comfortable by joking about my lost tresses. I said, "Hey, at least I have more than you!" I then grabbed a hunk from my head and it promptly fell out, right in my hand. I swear, he looked like he was going to faint. I laughed so hard that I pulled off some of the apparatuses that were hooked to the monitor from my chest. This was a disaster. The machine went haywire and flat-lined. All of these buzzers started going off, and nurses and doctors came running in. I was having the time of my life. You should have seen the look on my brother's face—it was classic.

Finally, I was released from my little glass prison. I went home with cropped hair. It was easier to manage it this way; every time I moved, more would fall out. I had to keep the windows shut in the car because my hair kept blowing off and out the window. I didn't care; I was so happy to go home.

When I arrived, my three best friends were waiting for me. They made me aware that I had to deal with my hair. We decided to visit the local barber and have him shave it off completely. When we got there, I told the guy to shave it off and don't dare ask why. I proceeded to turn my chair away from the mirror and watched the last of my mane fall to the floor. I did not even look when he was finished. I just got up and went home with my friends.

It took a long time for me to peek at my appearance. I had to convince myself that my new shiny head was "in vogue." The time came when I did catch a glimpse of myself in the mirror. I will never forget the feeling of my insides sinking down at the realization of my dreadful appearance. Besides my dazzling bald head, I had begun to show the effects of prednisone in my body. I gained 60 pounds and acquired a moon face without the benefits of eyebrows or eyelashes. You would think that, at least, the hair on my legs would have fallen out. Think again—it grew like weeds.

Throughout my trauma, I was numb. I bought a baseball hat with a naughty word on it and dealt with the loss of my hair the best way I could. I even went to a Sinead O'Connor concert. I needed to be with my kind. What a joke; I was made fun of twice. Those morons thought I was trying to imitate their leader. I went home from the show, downcast and sullen. To top off the whole brilliant night of fools and music, I took a shower and watched my pubic hair fall down the drain. It was then and there that I fully realized what was actually happening. For the very first time, my defenses melted, and I cried my eyes out.

My lovely high school was more than a bit sheltered; something like a student getting cancer was unheard of. I was the talk of the school. No one would ask me about my illness, and even though I was not in school, I heard all of the gossip. I had people from my class, who I was not even acquaintances with, just stop over to see "the girl with cancer." I felt like a one-woman sideshow. Even my best friend could not deal with my illness. It took her more than six months to come around and say hello. I was out of school and alone in my senior year. This was the year that everyone dreamed about since they were lowly freshmen. I was supposed to be going to parties, dances, and the prom.

I was home-tutored for most of the school year and had zero social life. Though I was not the type to really hit the dances, I was ill and really felt the need to experience some semblance of normalcy. I certainly could not get a date for any of the dances, so when my friend got her wits about her and came for a visit, she took me to the mall. We were going to the dances no matter what. We went looking for a dress, and I became so tired that she had to get me into a wheelchair. Wouldn't you know it, but the most popular group of boys came walking straight toward us as she wheeled me along. They crossed to the opposite side, carefully, so as not to make eye contact with me. These guys knew me but chose not to talk to or even look at me.

I did get to go to dances. My brother and a friend had asked some of their friends to escort me as favors. Of course, at the dances everyone kept their distance from the sick girl.

Boys were the only thing on my mind, besides my failing appearance. As I pined over love and the lack of it, I wrote this terrible poetry, wishfully thinking about the one guy who could see through this mask and . . . ? I never really dwelled on whether I would die, but I sure hoped I would get to "do it" before I did.

I was very lucky that I had a marvelous support team such as my friends. Everyone in my life at this period owns my heart. I will never forget the strength of everyone who put up with my frustrations and temper.

To be honest with you, it was never easy. It does hurt, emotionally and physically. Through it all, I must say that I learned about life the hard way. No one ever said life was fair, and this is the truth. The lessons I learned throughout "the cancer years" are etched into my soul like a slow-moving film. I can tell you just this: I am neither perfect nor superhuman, yet I made it. Do you want to live through this? Well, then do it and come tell me about it. I will be waiting.

Nikki Mosier

Type of cancer: Neuroblastoma
Age at diagnosis: 3
Current age: 15
Occupation: Student
Nikki's advice: You are not alone. There are tons of people out there who would do anything for you. Don't look at it as the end but rather as a beginning.

Nikki's Cancer Journey

I am 15 years old, and I survived cancer. When I was three, I was diagnosed with neuroblastoma. My tumor was in my neck. I was taken to Children's Hospital in Omaha, NE, where I was treated with chemotherapy and radiation for about three years. I lost my hair, but it didn't bother me because I was so young. I didn't understand exactly what was happening to me, yet I remember an awful lot about it.

While I was in the hospital, I met some extraordinary kids and wonderful nurses. I also met my best friend, Michelle, when I was five. That same year, I started going to Camp CoHoLo, a children's cancer camp in Gretna, NE. Michelle also went. CoHoLo stands for Courage, Hope, and Love. Doctors and nurses, as well as a great group of volunteers, are on site the whole time camp is in session. The camp started in 1985 with only a handful of campers and has grown so big that campers now are split into groups according to age. Many of the campers become counselors when they are old enough. Some people may look at cancer as the end, but my friends from camp and I look at it as the beginning. I wouldn't trade them for the world. I've met some of the most important people of my life through having cancer, and I'd never change it.

I'm now a sophomore in high school. Just by looking at me, you would never know that I had cancer. My hair has grown back and is down to the middle of my back. I can do anything anybody else can do. I'm very active in sports and extracurricular activities. Basketball is my all-time favorite.

I'm proud to tell people that I am a cancer survivor. I want to volunteer at Children's Hospital when I get to college and, someday, maybe even go into the medical field and help kids with cancer.

I never would have made it if it weren't for my parents and friends. Their love and support was more than I could have asked for. My sickness was really hard on them, but they never stopped supporting me. I wouldn't be where I am today without them.

Dominic Ramsey

Type of cancer: Non-Hodgkin's lymphoma
Age at diagnosis: 17
Current age: 28
Occupation: Web designer
Dominic's advice: Stay positive. Talk about how you are feeling.

Dominic's Cancer Journey

In 1987, when I was 17, I developed non-Hodgkin's lymphoma. At the time, I had never heard of lymphoma and had no idea what it meant or how it could affect me.

To better understand my experience with lymphoma, it is necessary to know a bit about my medical history. I was born without abdominal muscles and with poor kidney function. My left kidney was removed when I was very young, and over the years my right kidney progressively deteriorated. When I was 13, I had a kidney transplant. My father donated one of his kidneys, which was a good match and basically transformed my life.

All transplant recipients are given immunosuppressive drugs after a transplant to help to prevent the transplanted organ from being rejected. The drawback of this is that it makes a person with a transplant more susceptible to other illnesses because it depresses the immune system. If the person does get an illness, it is harder to fight off. This is probably why I developed lymphoma. Although I wasn't told about this at the time of my transplant, I later found out that lymphomas are quite common among transplant recipients who are taking immunosuppressants.

The first symptoms I experienced were fevers and night sweats. I didn't think much of it at the time because I didn't have particularly high temperatures, and the symptoms came on quite slowly. As usual, I delayed talking to the doctors about it, partly because I thought it was probably just the flu and partly because I was scared of what it might be. Around this time, I also had developed scoliosis, which is a curvature of the spine. I was starting to hate hospitals because it seemed like I was spending half of my life in them.

When I did go to the hospital, I was told that I had some type of fever, was given some medication, and was then told to go home. However, my night sweats got progressively worse and I couldn't sleep at night.

I again went to the hospital and underwent more tests. A lymph gland was removed from my neck. It was at this point that I was first told that I had lymphoma. I didn't have any idea what lymphoma was. When one of the doctors told me that it was similar to leukemia, I realized how serious it was.

The first thing that the doctors did was to stop the immunosuppressants in an attempt to boost my immune system. I knew that cutting out the antirejection drugs would not be good for my transplanted kidney, but everything was happening so quickly, and I didn't consider what the consequences of this might be.

A couple of weeks later, I started to feel nauseous and my hands and feet became swollen. More tests showed that the kidney had been rejected. I think I probably was more upset by this than when I was told that I had lymphoma. I knew it meant I would have to go on dialysis, and things just seemed to be getting worse and worse. I had a small operation to insert a tube for dialysis in the top of my leg. This was only a temporary measure, but it meant that I had to stay in the hospital and was not allowed to get out of bed until a more permanent access device could be inserted.

The lymphoma had not shown any signs of improvement, so I started a course of chemotherapy. The first injections didn't make me feel any different, other than mild nausea on the day of the injection. Over the course of the treatment, the side effects became more severe; my hair started to fall out and I became very depressed. This was just another side effect of the treatment rather than a reaction to my situation. The depression probably was the worst part of my whole experience with lymphoma. I didn't feel suicidal in any way, but I couldn't see any future, and I had lost the power to do anything.

Throughout the treatment, I had regular scans, which began to show some improvement. The last injection came as a relief, and it was clear that things were improving. The side effects of the drugs began to wear off. I started to feel normal again. Each scan showed another small improvement, and I began to look to the future. I had a dialysis machine installed at home, which meant I could begin to lead a normal life again. Soon, I was told I was "clear."

I continued to undergo dialysis at home for six years, and then the doctors decided it would be safe for me to have another kidney transplant. I was put on a waiting list, and within two weeks, I had a new kidney.

I'm back on immunosuppressants and at risk of getting lymphoma again. It was a difficult decision to make, but not being tied to a dialysis machine three times a week means my life is back to normal. I have problems with my joints, which are caused by the large doses of steroids that I received both during chemotherapy and after the transplants, but it's a small price to pay.

Andrea Richardson

Type of cancer: Acute myeloblastic leukemia
Age at diagnosis: 8; relapsed at age 12
Current age: 20
Occupation: Childcare worker with kids who have disabilities or who are chronically ill
Andrea's advice: Don't focus on all of the bad. Realize that cancer can be a blessing, as it can teach you what is important in life. It can make you a stronger person and can bestow upon you a profound appreciation for life.

Andrea's Cancer Journey

As a young child, I had a life that was as close to perfect as possible. I had two loving parents and a little sister, and I lived in a nice house in the suburbs of Washington, DC. I went to a good school, and on the weekends, I rode my bike and played soccer with my friends. It was a life in which bad things were not supposed to happen.

I was in the third grade when everything changed. It began with a few bruises on my legs and then a sore throat and fever that just wouldn't go away. My mother was concerned because I never got sick. She took me to the doctor. The doctor assured us that it was probably nothing more than an infection, but he ordered some tests "just to be sure." Three days after that initial visit to the doctor, I was in the hospital, being told that I had cancer.

"You have something called acute myeloblastic leukemia," the doctor said. My parents and I sat there dumbstruck. I remember sitting between my parents, listening to the doctor describe this disease that I had. As he talked about white blood cells, red blood cells, and blasts, I looked past him and down to the trees that lined the street below. As he described the chemotherapy drugs that were going to be used to fight the cancer in my body, I noticed how pretty all the gold, red, and orange leaves were. As the doctor talked about side effects and statistics, I realized that these same pretty leaves were going to be dead in just a few weeks.

When I was first diagnosed, I did not believe that I had cancer. I thought that I was going to wake up and discover that it was all a dream. I would pray to God every night before I went to sleep and ask Him to just let me wake up back in my own house the next morning and not be in a hospital room where I had to face cancer and chemotherapy. This never happened.

Each day I would get massive doses of chemotherapy. Words like *cytarabine, daunorubicin,* and *etoposide* became embedded in my vocabulary. Unlike my classmates, who were learning their multiplication tables and how to write in cursive, I was learning how to withstand the pain of bone marrow aspirations and spinal taps and how to flush my central line and give myself intramuscular injections.

I often would ask my mother why God let me get cancer, and she always would try to help me to find some comfort in the situation. She would remind me that bad things can be good, as they teach you about life and help you to uncover a strength that will help you to get through anything. I would contemplate her words, letting them roll around in my mind when I was too tired or sick to talk, wondering constantly what good was going to come out of me having cancer.

It wasn't until I began to feel better that I found some good in the situation. When I was finally able to return to school, I realized that cancer had made me different. Some of the differences I did not like. I hated it when people talked about my bald head or why I was always absent. I hated it when kids teased me or when teachers hovered around me, always asking if I was okay or if I could do this or that. I also realized, however, that I knew things that the other kids did not know. I appreciated life much more than they seemed to. Suddenly, the littlest things in life brought me the greatest happiness. I was content to just see a pretty sunset or hold a little baby. I knew this greater gratitude for things in life was the positive side of me having leukemia.

After I was in remission, my life slowly began to get back to normal. As the chemotherapy came in less frequent intervals, I began to get stronger. My hair grew back, and I regained lost weight. In the fall of 1990, four years after I found out that I had leukemia, I was starting the seventh grade. To look at me, you never would have known that I had cancer, and the whole experience was beginning to seem like a distant memory. With the excitement of starting junior high, I didn't even notice that something was wrong. First it was the occasional bruise that I chalked up to gym class, and then there was the fatigue, which I attributed to just getting up earlier to catch the bus, but as these symptoms became worse, I grew concerned. In the back of my mind, I knew that the cancer had returned.

That November, we were again sitting in the doctor's office being told that I had relapsed. It was a lot like the first time I learned that I had cancer. Once again, I looked past the doctor and out to the trees below, watching the leaves take on the autumn colors. Once again, I thought, This cannot be happening to me.

It also was different from the first time I was told that I had cancer.

At this point in my life, my doctor was like an old friend. I noticed tears in his eyes as he told me that I had relapsed. Unlike the first time, when I knew nothing of what was ahead of me, I now knew. I was now well immersed in the world of cancer. I knew that little could be done for a relapse of my type of leukemia, and this time, instead of thinking of the leaves that were dying outside, I was thinking of my own death.

I was told that a bone marrow transplant was my best option for beating the cancer, and even though my little sister was a five out of six match as a marrow donor for me, my best chance of surviving was still less than 10%. The bone marrow transplant was totally optional. I was given the choice of going through the bone marrow transplant or going home to die. I decided to try the transplant.

I went into the process with a positive attitude. I was fighting because I was determined to live. I had to sign a consent form before the process began, and my mother and I took the form home to read over the protocol and all of the possible side effects. The list seemed to go on forever. It talked of the routine side effects from chemotherapy and radiation, such as baldness, nausea, fatigue, and mouth sores. I had experienced all of these effects the first time around. Other things on this list I never had to deal with before. The forms discussed infertility, and at the age of 12, I had to deal with the fact that, if I were to live, I wouldn't be able to have children of my own. I read about possible blindness, deafness, paralysis, fatal heart damage, brain damage, and death. It felt too overwhelming to deal with, but I knew it was something that I had to do. My mother and I signed the consent form and returned it to the doctor. I felt as if I had just signed my life away.

The process for the transplant began, and I went into an isolation room to protect against the constant threat of infection. Intense chemotherapy and radiation not only killed the cancer that lurked in my bone marrow, but it also ravaged my immune system. I remember laying there, receiving chemotherapy one day, realizing that I couldn't turn back. It was the transplant or death. I prayed to God to let it work, to let me once again be able to live a normal life, a life free of cancer.

On April 11, 1991, my little sister was taken into the operating room, where marrow was extracted from her hip. The healthy bone marrow was brought to me, where I lay waiting in isolation for a second chance at life. The marrow contained in a bag was red, but it seemed to shimmer like gold. To me, it was full of life. I watched as the nurse carefully hooked up the bag of bone marrow to my central line. I watched as the marrow dripped down into the tube, where it mixed with the IV solution, turning from a bright red to a cloudy orange substance. I waited, and my mother, dressed in green scrubs, a mask, and gloves, held my hand. I imagined the healthy red and white cells filling up my bone marrow, making me stronger. I imagined getting better.

The post-transplant road was a long and scary one. It was filled with twists, turns, and sometimes what seemed like avalanches. My blood counts would go up, only to plummet the next day. I would develop mysterious infections and fevers and a case of graft-versus-host disease, which almost killed me. More than two months passed before I was stable enough to be moved out of isolation. Finally, almost four months after I was first admitted to the hospital for my bone marrow transplant, I was going home.

That was seven years ago. I am 20 years old now and a college student. Some days I wake up in the morning in utter disbelief that I have made it as far as I have. It has by no means been an easy journey. For the first three years after the transplant, managing the side effects from the treatment that I had undergone was difficult. I always will have to live under a cloud, knowing that I could either experience fatal side effects from my treatment, have another relapse, or develop a secondary cancer.

I would trade none of the pain that cancer has caused me for any of the splendid gifts that cancer has given me. Because of what I have been through, I take nothing in this world for granted. I am thankful for every breath, every flower, every sunset. I no longer think about the things that I have missed out on or may never get to do because of having had leukemia, but I think about the things that I have done. I have made some great friends and learned some valuable lessons about life. I have learned not to be afraid of death and to just appreciate the time that I have. I've acquired the ability to treasure every precious second of life.

Julia Ann (nee Smakula) Ryan

Type of cancer: Parotid gland mucoepidermoid carcinoma
Age at diagnosis: 11
Current age: 37
Occupation: Geriatric LPN/medical transcriptionist
Julia's advice: I think it helps to be a calm and cooperative patient. Make room in your mind and heart only for positive thoughts and feelings. Keep your faith and let it be strengthened. (I was diagnosed with a high-grade malignancy in 1973 and was not expected to survive. The medical field is so much more advanced today than it was 25 years ago.) Love is the greatest source of strength and healing. A sense of humor can be very helpful. Keep your heart light.

Julia's Cancer Journey

I spent my 12th birthday in the Children's Hospital of Philadelphia. I am now 37 years old and have not met one other person over the past 25 years who has a history of parotid gland cancer as a child.

Heidi Barone Sanford

Type of cancer: Wilms' tumor
Age at diagnosis: 13
Current age: 24
Occupation: Social worker
Heidi's advice: Have an enormous amount of faith in Jesus. A positive attitude will make a remarkable difference in your recovery. Stay close to your loved ones, and remember that even if you are diagnosed with a dreadful disease, miracles happen, and I am an example of that.

Heidi's Cancer Journey

I was diagnosed with Wilms' tumor at the age of 13. One day I began to notice a pain in my left side, especially when I would lie down or sit up. During gym class, I started to feel more pain than ever before. I told the teacher that I didn't feel well and asked to be excused that day. He did not allow that, and I felt very angry with him. When I got home from school, I told my mom I had a sharp pain in my side, and she suggested we go to the emergency room.

I went through a number of tests that night and then was sent to a hospital in Syracuse, NY, an hour away from where I live. I started to become more nervous as I went through more tests and probing. The doctors called us into a huge conference room, like the ones you see on television, to explain what was wrong. I looked over at my mom and asked her if I had cancer.

I had a tumor the size of a football wrapped around my kidney. They tried to take it out surgically, but they couldn't. I started chemotherapy and radiation treatments that lasted for a number of months and then had surgery again. They were unable to save my kidney. I continued treatment, and the following year, in the same month I was first diagnosed, the doctors discovered a lesion on my lung. They did not have to take any part of my lung. I started to receive a stronger type of chemotherapy every day for a week. I would then go home for two weeks and then return for another week-long stay at the hospital.

Keeping up with school work and dealing with some of my classmates was a challenge. One day at school, I pulled a hat off of a guy's head, and he responded by saying, "Leave me alone or I will pull your wig off." That didn't make having cancer any easier.

Before I started to lose my hair, it became very matted. My sister, who is eight years older than me, decided to help me to comb it. As she combed, it just started coming out. My mom, sister, and I cried the entire time she combed what was left of my hair. That was one of the most difficult times I went through.

Another time, one of my father's friends was staying with us, and I was called to dinner. I didn't realize that I didn't have my wig on. When I sat down at the table he said, "I didn't know that wasn't your real hair." I recall putting my hand on my head and noticing that my wig wasn't there.

My doctors told me that I wasn't going to live at the onset of the illness, so they were surprised to see me doing so well. I give all the credit to Jesus. I believe that He saved me, and that is the only reason I am alive. At the end of my second year of chemotherapy, I remember my doctor coming in to ask me if I would be excited about finishing my second year of chemotherapy. He joked around with me and told me that I was done after that stay in the hospital. I was so thrilled. I couldn't believe that the heartache, pain, and hospital stays were over.

I am now 24 years old and doing very well.

Annalee S. Tan

Type of cancer: Thyroid cancer
Age at diagnosis: 19
Current age: 20
Occupation: Medical student
Annalee's advice: Being diagnosed with a potentially fatal disease is hard enough. It's twice as difficult if you are a teenager who is old enough to have enjoyed a taste of life and yet young enough to have a lifetime ahead. It's tempting to wallow in depression and self-pity, but no one should ever give up. All the medicine and technology in the world can't help you if you have the wrong attitude.

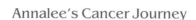

Annalee's Cancer Journey

It has become so routine that I hardly pay attention to it. I get out of bed, reach for two bottles on my dresser, take one pill from each bottle, and then get back into bed for an hour. After the alarm clock rings for a second time, I start the everyday routine that normal people go through: take a shower, eat breakfast, brush my teeth, get into my uniform, and rush over to class for my first lecture.

Yes, I have two wake-up times. After taking my medicine, I'm not allowed to eat for an hour. I can't take pills after breakfast because they have to be taken on an empty stomach. It took me quite a while to get used to taking my medicine under the right circumstances. For a few weeks, I went to school without breakfast because I had forgotten to take my medicine as soon as I woke up. A friend of mine devised the two-alarm-clock scheme, and I liked it.

I was 19 when I was diagnosed with thyroid cancer. I was in my last semester of premedical schooling, and I was preparing for my first semester of medical school. Talk about pressure. To make matters worse, the diagnosis came just days before registration. My thyroid had to come out. Suddenly, I was faced with a crucial decision—have the operation and miss the first few weeks of school or wait four months until our semester break and have the operation then. I opted to wait.

When I came to school, I faced a myriad of reactions from classmates and friends. People began to treat me like an invalid—friends carried my unbelievably heavy books; they made sure I wasn't alone when I walked to my dorm; and if I was a mere 10 minutes late, my pager would start beeping. The attention was flattering, but it was getting annoying. After all, it wasn't as if I had been handed an immediate death sentence.

That semester, I threw myself into my studies and extracurricular activities. The only outward sign that I was ill was a sign on my refrigerator that read, "Don't eat until you've taken your medication." I didn't need to be reminded. The thyroid is the organ responsible for metabolism, and if I ever forgot to take my pills (which are synthetic hormones), side effects like sleepiness, sluggishness, and mental laziness certainly would teach me a lesson.

Those four months went by with a blur of activity, and suddenly it was time for my operation. My scientific training seemed to crumble. I was so scared. I began to cry in the waiting room. I guess I still wasn't the stoic doctor I was studying to become but rather a scared little girl.

They say that doctors make the worst patients. I think the same holds true for first-year medical students. Every time something felt weird, I'd bug the nurses and residents, asking if something could have gone wrong with some nerve they might have hit during the surgery. Then there was the experience of having the stitches removed. My imagination went haywire thinking of all the possible scenarios: a nerve caught on a thread, an infection settling in once the stitches were gone, some of the thread getting stuck and becoming a permanent component of my neck. I learned something that our patient-relationship classes never taught us: how a patient really feels.

When I went back for my second semester of medical school, the scar on my neck became a source of interest to some of my classmates and teachers. Still, I refused to dwell on the fact that I had just had major surgery. I focused most of my energy on my studies and on extracurricular activities. As I ran from meeting to meeting, or pulled all-nighters before an exam, people shook their heads in disbelief. I was just a few weeks out of the recovery period and running around nonstop. I was exhausted, but I couldn't bring myself to stop. To do so would be to admit that the cancer had won. And no patient should ever be allowed to admit that.

So I went about the normal patterns of my daily life. Books, meetings, experiments, research papers, and occasional trips to the mall. The only thing different was that I had to get up an hour earlier than usual to take my medication.

One of my claims to fame is that I never missed a day of high school or college. Two months after my operation, I cut my morning lecture. I had to go to the hospital to have a scan done to check and see if there was any residual tissue thyroid left. As much as I had hoped that the scan would show nothing, the film showed something that even a first-year medical student could understand: the surgery did not remove all of the thyroid tissue and there was still a chance of my cancer recurring. Two weeks before Christmas, my doctor advised that I undergo radiation therapy.

As far as school was concerned, January was one of the lightest months in terms of exams and projects. My doctor told me that I had to be isolated for three days, depending on how fast the radiation cleared from my body. I practically threw a tantrum in his office. There was no way that I was going to miss three days of school, no matter how boring the week was going to be. In the end, however, he won out. I entered the hospital on the week of my 20th birthday.

That week was one of the worst of my life. I threw up. I couldn't eat. I spent half of the day on the toilet. I couldn't see anybody. I had headaches and was sick to my stomach. No matter what type of medicine I took, the side effects wouldn't go away. I also had an exam at the end of the week. Happy Birthday to me.

Six weeks later, I was back at the hospital. I had cut another morning lecture and was undergoing another scan to see if the radiation destroyed the residual tissue. This time, I didn't see the film. I had to wait a week to find out the results.

Luckily, for my sanity, I had about six exams to study for that week. I didn't let myself dwell on the possible results of the scan; I spent the week studying like crazy. The night before the last exam of that week, I found out that the scan revealed no remaining thyroid tissue. I had just won the battle.

I knew I was in for a tough time when I got accepted into medical school, but I never expected to have been personally confronted with cancer during my first year. As I enter my second year of medical school, a year that is supposedly the toughest, I know that I have a slight advantage over most of my classmates. I will know what it feels like to not yet be legally an adult and yet be threatened by cancer, the "plague of the 20th century." I will know how it feels to have stitches removed. I will know the fears a patient hides from his or her doctor. I will know how dependent a patient is on anything his or her doctor says and does. I will know never to give up, despite how many obstacles are placed in front of me.

I have been on both sides of the doctor-patient relationship. I hope that all of these lessons that can never be taught, only experienced, will help me to become a better doctor. While a patient's physical well-being is dependent upon the medicine and technology that scientific research can uncover, the patient's total well-being depends much on support, determination, understanding, and the love that is given. Only when a successful harmony is achieved can the war be won.

Maria Valarezo

Type of cancer: Acute lymphoblastic leukemia (ALL)
Age at diagnosis: 13
Current age: 20
Occupation: Full-time student, part-time library aid
Maria's advice: Be strong, but allow yourself to cry. Part of being strong is knowing when to cry. Furthermore, find someone you can really talk to.

Maria's Cancer Journey

I was filled with fear when I was told that I had leukemia. I was 13 years old. I was in a hospital bed, recovering from a bone marrow biopsy that was performed earlier that day. Now it was evening, and my mother and I were waiting for the doctor to come by on his evening rounds so that he could tell us the results.

My mind was consumed with all sorts of scenarios about what was going wrong inside my body. I hoped and prayed that the diagnosis would not be serious. The prospect of being seriously ill terrified me.

After what seemed like forever, the doctor came in and asked to speak to my mother. I felt afraid and alone. My mother and the doctor came back into the room. The air inside the room became still as the doctor prepared to tell me the news. It seemed as if time stopped for that moment. Suddenly, the stillness was shattered by the blaring ring of the telephone. I ignored it and demanded that the doctor tell me what was wrong with me. My heart was pounding. Soon my nightmare became a reality as my doctor told me that I had cancer. I asked him, "Where is my cancer?"

He replied, "Do you know where your blood is?"

I said, "All over."

He said, "That is where your cancer is."

Fear came over me, and I blocked out everything else the doctor was saying. The idea of a child, me, having cancer was hard to swallow. I felt like I was falling into a black abyss. I became haunted by terrifying thoughts of death that infiltrated my mind.

And so I began my two-and-one-half year fight for life—a fight that I won. Leukemia has taught me to always have faith, no matter what.

Brett Wilson

Type of cancer: Acute lymphoblastic leukemia and non-Hodgkin's lymphoma
Age at diagnosis: 2 (with leukemia) and 9 (with lymphoma)
Current age: 26

Occupation: Cancer counselor, Long-Term Survivors Program at Duke University
Brett's advice: Trust in God as hard as it may seem. Never give up, and keep a positive attitude.

Brett's Cancer Journey

In 1974, when I was two years old, I was diagnosed with leukemia. I started chemotherapy and endured it for five years. I hardly remember much about this time because I was so young, but my mother tells me that I was very sick. My leukemia, however, did go into remission.

After I beat leukemia, I went in for routine checkups. During one of the checkups seven years after my first diagnosis, my doctor said that I had non-Hodgkin's lymphoma. I just broke down crying and asked, "Why me?"

My treatment for lymphoma involved both chemotherapy and radiation. The worst part of it was laying on the cold table in the radiation room. I would look at the X and feel the heavy metal shield pressing against my chest. Sometimes I would become so bored that I would fall asleep.

Once while I was undergoing a CT scan, I became terrified because there was a woman patient in the room who just lay on a stretcher, wrapped in a sheet. I thought she was dead, and I totally flipped out. I soon found out, however, that she was just cold so the technician had given her sheets to help warm her.

I hated going to school because everyone would tease me and make fun of me. The radiation and chemotherapy caused me to lose my hair, and I gained so much weight that I had to wear big clothes. Fortunately, my older brother and his friends stuck by me.

I loved science and gym, but all through grade school, junior high, and high school I had problems with math. During high school, I discovered that I had some real learning difficulties. I would study for hours, memorize and repeat the information, and still fail the tests. Finally, I was tested in college and found out I had symptoms of attention deficit disorder. I experienced problems staying focused for long periods of time and had test anxiety. These symptoms were coupled with short-term memory loss. I did learn how to overcome my disabilities. I worked hard, was determined and willing, and went to a tutoring program. Eventually, I earned a master's degree in counseling.

Cancer has changed me in many ways. I feel like a 40-year-old in a 25-year-old body. I'm now aware of my own mortality. I don't worry about things I cannot control because I find no point in it. I also find great joy in helping other people because I know what it feels like to be a person who is not helped.

I believe that people can survive cancer and lead productive lives. I certainly have.

Your Cancer Journey

Where will your journey take you?

Chapter 9.

The End, but Not Really: The Journey Continues

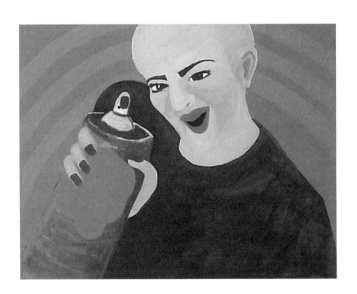

Chapter 9.

The End, but Not Really: The Journey Continues

I think there was a part of me, a very small part of me, that decided to go into a year-intense master of education program, which includes a teaching certification in grades 1 through 8, because I knew it would be physically grueling and I needed to prove to myself that I could do it. My biggest fear was that my physical limitations would make me an inadequate teacher or prohibit me altogether from becoming a teacher. No matter how hard I tried to convince myself that I was, indeed, capable and adequate, I couldn't shake my fear.

It's amazing how I was mentally defeated before I even started the program. Ironically, I didn't have to look far to see an example of someone who overcame a physical disability to go on and become an extraordinary teacher. My favorite math teacher in high school is legally blind. She once told me that when she was a child, some ignorant person told her mother that she would probably have to make her living selling pencils. Instead, she went to college and graduate school. She was the best math teacher I ever had.

As the year started, I was student-teaching during the day and taking graduate classes at night. There were days when my legs would give out. At the end of the day, when I was walking to the car, I was using walls to help to support my walking. I wasn't going to use my crutches because, in my mind, that would mean that I was giving in.

I constantly worried that my students would say something about the way I walked. Occasionally, one of the students would ask, and then another would ask a few weeks later, and so on. I'd explain that I had a problem with my legs because I was sick a long time ago and that I was still healing. They were always kind, and some would ask how I was feeling on any particular day.

A few weeks later, I noticed that one of the boys in my class was watching me, studying me walk. I observed him observing me because I found that the children were curious about why I walked the way I walked, but they were never cruel. So I watched this nine-year-old watch me for about three months.

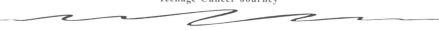

And then picture day came.

I was supervising the students as they stood in line after they got their pictures taken. As it happened, I was standing right in front of the student who was watching me walk. I could feel what was about to happen.

"Miss Gill, I've been watching you walk," he said.

Feeling hesitant, I replied, "Oh, you have been, have you?"

"Yeah, I've been trying to walk like you," he said.

I must admit, I was puzzled. So I asked him, "Why?"

"I want to know how you do it. When I try it, my foot really hurts," he said.

I just looked at him and smiled. Here I was, totally self-conscious about the way I walked, and one of my students wasn't imitating me in a mocking way, but rather trying to figure out how I could pull off such a neat trick.

I made it into November, and then I crashed. I couldn't physically go on with the program. I was experiencing this horrible burning sensation in my legs, and the pain was intense and constant. I was so stiff that I had to roll myself out of bed and onto the ground every morning. Then, I'd get into the shower and my joints slowly would start to loosen under the intense heat of the scalding water. I also was beating myself up. I felt like a total failure, personally and professionally. I hated who I had become. I had become my worst fears.

I think one of the hardest things I ever had to do was explain to my class of eight- and nine-year-olds why I had to leave them. Basically, I said that I had a problem with my hip (most of them knew about that by now, anyway) and that I had to take some time off to get better and maybe have surgery. I remember biting into my cheek to keep myself from crying in front of them.

I completed the remainder of my graduate classes at home. I'm not even sure how I did that. I sank into a deep depression. I was sad and angry. I cried constantly. I slept.

I felt like a complete and total failure. I felt that no one could possibly understand. I felt that it would be easier to give up entirely on my master's degree and on teaching. I tried to convince myself that teaching wasn't for me. I just couldn't see a way that it would all work out. Thankfully, people in the elementary school where I was working and at my university wouldn't let me give up so easily.

Within a few weeks, everything was worked out. I would come back and complete my degree and teaching certification the following year. My one job for the next nine months was to get better. This involved getting better not only physically but also mentally and emotionally.

I don't think I ever grieved over how my life had changed after having cancer. I never stopped to think about the situation with my hips. Instead, I ignored it. This worked in high school and college because I got around on crutches and told elaborate stories about how I injured myself. But now, I needed to deal with how I was going to adapt and make it in the world.

I worked hard physically and grew stronger. I now take better medication and wear lifts in my shoes to help to take pressure off of my legs when I walk. I never would have done that last year because I thought that it meant that I was weak. Now I look at it as doing what I have to do in order to accomplish my goal of becoming a teacher. I also accept help and adapt to classroom situations by staggering times when I sit and times when I stand.

I also know that no matter what happens this year, I will complete my program and finish my year of student teaching. I know this because I will come in a wheelchair if I have to, and I know that I am the only one I have to convince that this will not be a problem. I have many of the same students in class that I had last year. I plan on sitting down with them and discussing my cancer experience with them. While it is important to teach them reading, math, science, spelling, language, and social studies, I feel that it is equally important to teach them that hard things happen in life and that people can get through them. I also want their perception of cancer to be different. I want them to see that people can get over cancer and go on with their lives.

I am constantly reminded of perspective. It's like the time my student didn't see that I had a problem walking but rather thought I was pulling off an amazing trick. And so I'll conclude by saying that being given the opportunity to write this book is one of best opportunities I have ever been given, and I owe its existence to one of the worst things, possibly the worst thing, that ever happened to me.

Chapter 10.

Tips I Picked Up Along the Way

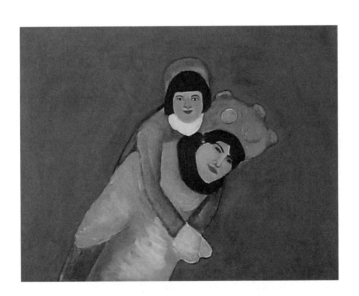

Chapter 10.

Tips I Picked Up Along the Way

As I traveled along, sometimes crawling, on my own cancer journey, I took notes about certain insights I had at different times. The following list resulted from one of my long hospital stays.

On Hospitals

1. Bring your own clothes, pajamas, robe, and slippers. You always feel better in your own stuff than in those hospital gowns.
2. When you feel decent, have your friends come to visit or call them on the phone.
3. If you're not feeling well or don't feel like visiting, pretend that you are asleep.
4. If you feel like you're going to go crazy in your hospital room and you can't stand to be in there a minute longer, take a trip down to the nursery and look at the babies.
5. Bring CDs, a radio, books, and other random stuff from home to keep you busy.
6. Ask your doctor for an estimate of how long you'll be in. I used to forget that I would eventually get out of the hospital.
7. Tap into the hospital's resources—lending library, video games, and VCRs.
8. Make small talk with your nurses—hospitals are full of interesting stories. I also have found that a stay is more pleasant once you get the nurses on your side.

I took note as certain issues arose with my friends. Here are some of my thoughts.

On Friends

1. Remember they cannot read your mind.
2. When you're feeling left out, tell them. Don't make them guess what's wrong. That gets old fast.
3. They might not know what it's like to have cancer, but you don't know what it's like to have a friend with cancer.
4. Some friends might disappoint you with their reactions to your illness. Good

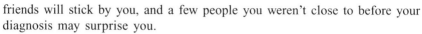

friends will stick by you, and a few people you weren't close to before your diagnosis may surprise you.

5. Sometimes when I was angry or just plain fed up, I used to say things for effect. Comments like "Well, you're going to have to find a new friend after I die" made my friends understandably feel uncomfortable.

6. Don't mistake not knowing what to say and staying away for a little while as not caring. Your friends need some time to process what is happening, too.

7. At times it might seem like your friends are on easy street. Remember, they are dealing with issues, too. It's not a "who is suffering more" contest.

8. Communicate, communicate, communicate!

9. Be honest with your friends and accept that they will be honest with you, too. Honesty may hurt.

Other Random Thoughts

1. Feelings are never wrong. There isn't one way to react to getting cancer.

2. Talk to people about your fears.

3. Anger is a powerful weapon. Be careful what you say in anger. Even if you apologize, it's hard to forget the sting of the words.

4. You are not always going to feel horrible, even though I know you may not believe this right now.

Available Resources

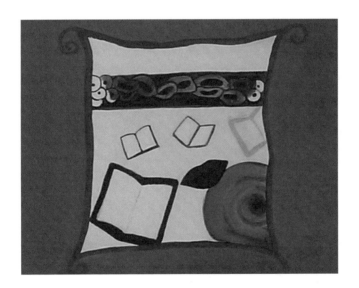

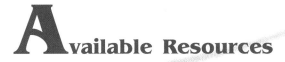

Available Resources

Books, Movies, and Music

Three of the best books I have ever read about cancer are the following.

1. *Autobiography of a Face,* by Lucy Grealy, 1994, Boston: Houghton Mifflin Company, 223 pages, $12.00

   This is a woman's account of her experience with Ewing's sarcoma. Her cancer was located in her jaw. Diagnosed as a preadolescent, Lucy endured years of chemotherapy and surgery. Lucy talks about her struggles for acceptance as the many surgeries left her face disfigured.

2. *I Want to Grow Hair, I Want to Grow Up, I Want to Go to Boise,* by Erma Bombeck, 1989, New York: Harper & Row, 144 pages, $16.95

   It's a book about children and young adults dealing with cancer. Trust me, you'll laugh.

3. *Comeback,* by Dave Dravecky, 1990, Grand Rapids, MI: Zondervan Publishing House, 252 pages, $8.99

   This is the story of San Francisco Giants pitcher Dave Dravecky and his struggle with cancer in his pitching arm.

Two of the best movies I have ever seen about cancer are the following.

1. *Dying Young*

   I know the title may not sound too promising, but you will be surprised by how the movie ends. This is a story of a young man, played by Campbell Scott, who has just suffered a relapse of his leukemia. Understandably, he is depressed. His wealthy father hires a beautiful caregiver, played by Julia Roberts, to help his son through this difficult time.

2. *The Doctor*

   William Hurt plays an arrogant surgeon who learns that he has throat cancer. His diagnosis and having to go through cancer treatment helps him to understand the patient side of illness.

The best cancer-related CD in my opinion is Kevin Sharp's *Measure of a Man.* Kevin Sharp, a country singer, had Ewing's sarcoma. He went on to beat it and fulfill his dream of becoming a successful country singer. Before I even heard about him or his story, I heard the song "Nobody Knows" and thought, "I bet the person who wrote that song had cancer."

Organizations to Contact

The Candlelighters Childhood Cancer Foundation publishes two newsletters. One is for adult survivors of childhood cancer, and the other is for children and young adults currently in treatment. These publications are free. This organization also offers other useful publications. Call 800-366-2223 for details.

The Leukemia Society of America offers services to people with leukemia, Hodgkin's disease, non-Hodgkin's lymphoma, and multiple myeloma. It offers a program that provides mileage and parking reimbursements and also offers many publications. Check the telephone book to locate your local chapter.

Vanderbilt Children's Hospital offers publications that deal specifically with cancer and younger people. They can be reached by calling 800-288-0391.

The Lynn Marcell Community Resource Center is one of only a handful of comprehensive cancer libraries in the United States. The resource librarian, Eileen Cohen, is a master at finding any materials you may need. Call 216-476-6949 for information.

The National Cancer Institute offers many free publications. They can be reached by calling 800-4-CANCER.

The American Cancer Society also offers many free publications. Call 800-227-2345.

The Internet

The Internet, with what seems like an unlimited amount of information, can be overwhelming. The following is a list of Web addresses that can guide you to cancer-related information from reputable sources. Many of the sites have additional links.

1. The National Children's Cancer Society: www.children-cancer.com/start.html
2. Oncolink®—University of Pennsylvania Cancer Center: www.oncolink.upenn.edu/
3. Cancer Kids: www.cancerkids.org
4. Leukemia Society of America: www.leukemia.org
5. American Cancer Society: www.cancer.org/
6. National Coalition for Cancer Survivors—Cansearch: www.cansearch.org/index.html
7. National Cancer Institute—Cancernet™: www.nci.nih.gov/
8. Memorial Sloan-Kettering Cancer Center: www.mskcc.org/
9. Dave's Happy Little Hodgkin's Web Site: www.davesite.com/hodgkins/
10. The Lymphoma Information Network: www.lymphomainfo.net/